THE
FIT
VEGAN

THE
FIT
VEGAN

Fuel Your Fitness with a
Plant-Based Lifestyle

EDRIC KENNEDY-MACFOY

HAY HOUSE

Carlsbad, California • New York City
London • Sydney • New Delhi

Published in the United Kingdom by:
Hay House UK Ltd, The Sixth Floor, Watson House,
54 Baker Street, London W1U 7BU
Tel: +44 (0)20 3927 7290; Fax: +44 (0)20 3927 7291
www.hayhouse.co.uk

Published in the United States of America by:
Hay House Inc., PO Box 5100, Carlsbad, CA 92018-5100
Tel: (1) 760 431 7695 or (800) 654 5126
Fax: (1) 760 431 6948 or (800) 650 5115; www.hayhouse.com

Published in Australia by:
Hay House Australia Ltd, 18/36 Ralph St, Alexandria NSW 2015
Tel: (61) 2 9669 4299; Fax: (61) 2 9669 4144; www.hayhouse.com.au

Published in India by:
Hay House Publishers India, Muskaan Complex,
Plot No.3, B-2, Vasant Kunj, New Delhi 110 070
Tel: (91) 11 4176 1620; Fax: (91) 11 4176 1630; www.hayhouse.co.in

A catalogue record for this book is available from the British Library.

ISBN: 978-1-4019-6039-1
E-book ISBN: 978-1-78817-098-7

Interior illustrations: Shutterstock

*To my Father, Thomas, for levelling up in every way
possible. You found the strength and courage to change
your mindset. You transitioned to a plant-based lifestyle
and, in doing so, changed your life.
You too are an ambassador for change.
Thank you for your love and guidance.
I feel blessed to have you in my life.*

Contents

The Fit Vegan Workout: List of Exercises

Introduction

Fit *and* Vegan

Fit and vegan. Two of my favourite words. To my mind, they go together like salt and pepper. Until a few years ago, along with many other people, I thought the opposite. The phrase 'vegan muscle' sounded like a bad joke. I was convinced that a healthy body needed to be fuelled with plenty of animal protein. I was a committed carnivore, with cupboards filled with milk-based protein shake mixes, and a fridge stuffed with chicken breasts, salmon fillets and lean beef. Fast forward a few years, and I've left all that behind me. My body is now stronger, leaner and fitter than ever before, and I nourish it with a whole food plant-based diet. As a result, I have more energy than ever and have noticed significant improvements in my mood, digestion and vitality.

I wanted to write this book to share my journey with you, revealing how and why you can switch to a plant-based lifestyle, and what to do to transform your body into a stronger, fitter, more sculpted, more flexible and more energized version of the one you currently have. I've spent years in the gym, training myself and others, initially as a bodybuilder and later as a personal trainer. I've learned how to get dramatic results in minimal time, and I've condensed that knowledge into a 12-week fitness plan for this book, which you can use for home- and gym-based workouts, and can be tailored to suit your body whatever level of fitness you're at right now.

I'll help you build your fitness as you develop your repertoire of delicious vegan meals, managing the transition from omnivorous or vegetarian, without the shock of cold turkey or the unsustainable faff of fiddly recipes with endless ingredients. I'll share the key facts and research I've uncovered as I've studied plant-based nutrition, on the course run by the vegan pioneer Dr Colin T Campbell at Cornell University, USA. I'll introduce you to fresh ingredients and reveal simple seasoning hacks to make your meals go from basic to brilliant.

I'll share some great places to eat out and tell you what to buy in the supermarket. I'll even help you work out what to say if friends, family or colleagues hit you with 20 questions about your new diet. When I went vegan, I was working as a firefighter in London, and I defy anyone to match the levels of interrogation disguised as banter I experienced there. I want to use my experience and newfound nutritional awareness to inspire you to have the confidence to make the change, saving you time in the gym and making sure you get more out of your workouts: results and fun.

Why now is a great time to go vegan

First up, I've got some good news. There has never been a better time to go vegan. Cutting out animal products no longer means compromising your social life, curtailing your adventurous and varied eating habits, or time-consuming and labour-intensive meal preparation. Restaurants have woken up to the demand for exciting vegan meals, most supermarkets have a plant-based range in addition to their fruit and veg aisle, and many cafés stock oat and almond milk alongside dairy. Veganism is having 'a moment', and that's great.

When I first transitioned, I found myself eating in my usual restaurants, with few or no vegan options to choose from. I'd often have to ask for a vegetarian dish to be made vegan, (or veganized as I've learned to call it) and this was sometimes met with sighs or flat-out refusals. It was painful: something I was once so fond of (eating out) had become an absolute bore. I sometimes felt self-conscious and awkward around friends. It's laughable now when I think about it because things have changed so much in such a short period. A little bit of research and a few years later, and most restaurants have caught up with their customer's requirements. I now have several firm vegan favourites. Even mainstream chain restaurants offer a few vegan options. Now it's rare to find restaurants without entire menus full of vegan, vegetarian, gluten-free, dairy-free and other types of dishes.

Vegan balance

Eating out aside, any sustainable dietary change needs to work on an everyday basis. And the key to a diet you can stick with is one that delights your taste buds and keeps you satiated, energized and nourished. In my quest to help clients tick all these boxes, I've spent a lot of time thinking about the poor eating habits that get in the way of achieving this balance, and how to avoid them. In particular, since I've been working as a nutrition and personal training consultant, I've noticed clients tend to fall into one of two camps when it comes to food. They either eat too much or not enough. Neither of these options is healthy. Overconsumption of food leads to excess fat and associated health issues, while an under-fuelled body won't have the energy to exercise and build muscle. Insufficient calories and nutrients mean mental clarity, agility and cognition are compromised too. I aim to help you provide the perfect ratio of nutrients and calories to give your body the energy it needs to fuel your workouts and your lifestyle. My meal plans are deprivation-free and keep effort and inconvenience to a minimum.

I hope the simplicity of The Fit Vegan (TFV) programme will make it ultra-easy to follow. This is because I recognize that it's all too easy to get into unhealthy habits when it comes to your diet, a fact that's equally applicable to vegans as it is of anyone following any type of diet or non-diet. So often, we seize on a random pick-and-mix of nutritional 'facts' and 'rules' without investigating them, and eat according to them, without assessing the evidence. We may continue adhering to these arbitrary principles for years, avoiding carbs because we once lost half a stone on the Atkins diet or spending a fortune on hard-to-source exotic superfoods because we think we need them.

Unhelpful dietary myths, such as 'carbs are bad for you', influence many of us. But lumping fries, white bread and biscuits in the same basket as sweet potatoes, brown rice and quinoa is crazy. Similarly, 'fats make you fat' is a vague, unhelpful statement that still has wide-reaching appeal. A battered sausage, for example, and an avocado are both high-fat foods, but they have little in common and any generalization implying they do is dangerous. To take a more logical approach, it's essential to have a basic understanding of macronutrients – what and how much our bodies need of the major food types, in particular, complex carbs and protein – I'll tackle this in Chapters 2 and 7.

As I've discovered on my vegan journey, it's worthwhile questioning all the 'facts' we've taken for granted about the healthiness of animal protein. Once you open yourself up to the possibility that animal products may not be the healthiest option, there's an overwhelming amount of nutritional research available to anyone who has the time and inclination to sift through it. I'll be drawing your attention to the persuasive research on veganism in the next few chapters, but one thing that struck me was the evidence from population-based 'epistemological' studies (a fancy word to describe studies that use large groups and populations and 'big data' correlations to map trends). Such studies, the most famous being 'The China Study', show that societies that consume the most animal products have the highest rates of bone fractures, osteoporosis and cancers. The same studies show the societies that consume little to no animal protein (Hindus, Jains, Seventh-day Adventists, Buddhists and Rastafarians) have lower incidences of these health issues.

Such studies get criticized because they don't prove a direct causal link (in contrast, a randomized controlled trial, known as the 'gold standard' for scientific research, would feed a test group of participants a set amount of meat every day then feed the other group a vegan diet, comparing the cancer incidence after ten years). Such research is scarce, and it's easy to see why because it would be almost impossible to control and police. But rather than dismissing epistemological evidence, a growing number of medical and dietary experts think we should sit up and take notice of what it's telling us. I'll leave you to draw your own conclusions, but the sheer scale of the numbers has me convinced.

My personal quest

I've had the first-hand experience of the devastation that 'lifestyle diseases' such as cancer and heart disease can have on families because they've torn through my own. In the past 15 years, I've lost my mother Rosemond, grandmother Isata Macfoy, Uncle Fred Macfoy, aunties Rosalyn Macfoy and Justina Sawyerr, cousin Donald McCormack and also countless friends, including two of my closest school friends to cancer, and in 2018 my father was diagnosed with prostate cancer. I don't require medical studies to see the causation between health and diet. I've seen and experienced it time and time again in my adult life. Without exception, all of the people I've lost were heavy consumers of animal products and processed meat.

When my mother was on her death bed, her cousin Dr Stella Cole, a general practitioner, was there the whole time supporting my family and talking to the medical professionals caring for my mother. But not once did she suggest it might be worth changing Mum's diet. I know from talking to Aunt Stella that dietary recommendations didn't occur to her because her medical training only sketchily touched on nutrition. Now, thanks to our dialogue, my aunt eats a predominantly plant-based diet.

Despite Aunt Stella's change of mind and the growing body of evidence linking major diseases with diet and lifestyle, conventional medicine still rejects a preventative approach. This seems so sad to me and so frustrating. Surely, we should learn about this stuff in school, and for sure, it should be a significant part of any doctor's training. I often ask myself:

'How many mothers, fathers, sisters and brothers will we have to lose before we decide that what we put in our bodies is so much more than taste, habit and convenience but matters to our health?'

Malaika's story

Let me tell you a story. In May 2018, I escaped to the USA for a long-awaited break after resigning from the fire service to spend some quality time with my family, mainly my favourite cousin Malaika Cherie. Before arriving, we'd had a few conversations in which she expressed an interest in learning more about plant-based nutrition and the vegan lifestyle. She'd been reading my Instagram posts and the material I was sharing relating to veganism and fitness – and unknown to me, it was resonating. Little did we know at the time but that unplanned last-minute trip to stay with Malaika would be the cause of a significant change in her life.

Excited about my arrival, Malaika saw the visit as her perfect opportunity to attempt to try out the vegan lifestyle. It would be simple. As she said when I first stepped into her family home, 'Yay, now that you're here, we're all going vegan. The whole family is going to eat what you're eating for the duration of your stay.'

And so, it began…

I kept it pretty simple: oats, quinoa or chia pudding for breakfast, a fruit and veg smoothie for a midmorning snack, and for lunch and dinner 50 per cent of the plate always consisted of a variety of vegetables while the remainder was a balance of essential macronutrients in the form of plant-based whole foods. Lucky for Malaika having a 'live-in chef' made the transition so much easier. We even veganized some of her favourite stews. We were also following my Fit Vegan fitness routine 5–6 mornings a week; we were feeling great and Malaika was feeling great. It was all good! I also upped Malaika's water intake, so she was drinking the recommended 2–3 litres (4–6 pints) per day.

Two months later Malaika pulled me aside; she had a look of relief on her face, and I could tell good news was on the horizon, but I'd no idea what it was. She told me her physician had found precancerous cells in her cervix three years ago, and she'd been attending the hospital every three months for check-ups ever since. Every three months for the past three years, the cells had progressively increased, and the doctors were now discussing surgical intervention. For three years, I'd been oblivious to this health issue, which had been weighing so heavily on her mind. So imagine her delight when she received a call following her first check-up after plant-based eating for two months. For the first time in three years, there had been a reduction in the precancerous cells. The one thing she'd changed was her diet. Although she wasn't struggling with this transition, this unbelievable improvement strengthened her 'why factor'. This was great news for me too, as I thought she'd slip back into eating animal products as soon as I returned to the UK. She didn't, and her journey continued.

Again, three months passed, and as Malaika waited for the latest results from the hospital, she wondered whether removing animal products from her diet had made the difference. The results came in, and for the second time in three years, there was a further reduction in these precancerous cells. So much so that the doctor changed her check-ups from quarterly to every six months. Again, Malaika continued with the plant-based eating and fitness routine.

Six months later, I received a call from Malaika. She told me she'd been struggling a little for the past few weeks and had just felt like eating some dairy. I questioned whether or not she went with that feeling. The answer was no. She then told me that the phone call from her doctor the day before had really put things in perspective because her cervix had returned to its normal healthy state. I believe, as does Malaika, that this improvement in her health issue is a testimony to the power of plant-based nutrition.

When Malaika decided to try the vegan lifestyle, she didn't stipulate the length of time she planned to eat this way. There was no pressure, only a willingness to learn and to try. Yet when Malaika visited Cancun for a week with her friends, she continued with a plant-based diet while watching her friends feast on foods she once loved – still loved, even though the vegan options were minimal. I was so impressed. And a year later, what had started off as 'I'll give this a try' was still in full swing. But she had another trip to the Dominican Republic fast approaching, and Malaika just felt like indulging. She missed cheese, her precise words were, 'It's a long time since I've had me some real cheese, I want to take a break from asking questions about the ingredients in the desserts, I just want to indulge.' She decided to adopt a vegetarian diet and to get her fill of dairy to satisfy her craving.

Day 1, cheese. Day 2, more cheese. And on day 3 her face broke out in pimples like never before. In 32 years, nobody had ever seen her face like that, she has amazing skin, and it was at its best after following a vegan diet for a year. She was distraught, but had to own the fact that she'd made a poor decision. It was only after this experience that Malaika realized just how toxic dairy was for her body. She said, 'My body seemed angry with my decision. When I went vegan, my body didn't go into shock and breakout.'

Malaika is now fully vegan and isn't looking back. Her Dominican Republic experience solidified everything for her. She was still hitting the gym really hard, practising yoga and remaining hydrated, but it wasn't enough. I found it fascinating how the body seems to cope with what we feed it. However, as soon as we take those toxins away, cleansing the system, then reintroduce them, the body puts up a fight. While you always need to seek help from your medical practitioner, there's no reason why food can't also be your daily medicine.

Vegan and black

Ethics and personal wellbeing aside, my remaining family is now one of my most significant motivating factors in maintaining a vegan lifestyle, especially my daughter, who is only seven years old. I feel a huge responsibility for her health. I have to own that and take it seriously. So how does being vegan benefit my family and me? I believe and hope that eating a nutritious vegan diet will help us to live longer, healthier and happier lives. It will help us to remain a family. I want to live to a happy old age. I want to enjoy my children, grandchildren and even great-grandchildren. As a man of colour with African and Caribbean heritage, I think it's important to highlight the importance and repercussions of our food choices, especially in the black community. People need to see others they can relate to, and I sincerely hope that in becoming a public spokesperson for the benefits of veganism, I'll make it more accessible for other vegans of colour.

Meat is a massive part of our culture. But to understand why African and Caribbean people find plant-based diets alien, it's essential to consider the cultural significance of meat. The roots of our attachments to eating animals run deep. If you look back to when people of colour were enslaved and oppressed, chicken, fish, pigs' trotters and other discarded animal parts were dietary staples. Our ancestors ate these foods in desperation, not because they were nutritious and healthy food choices. However, we've always been good at turning a negative into something positive, making the best of a bad situation, and so these staples were turned into various dishes and regarded as not just delicious, but a fundamental part of black culture. Now, the same food we ate to survive has been passed down generation to generation.

Before I contemplated veganism I viewed it as a white thing, simple as that. Anything vegan I heard of, and any vegans I met, were white. Even now, when veganism is more widespread and organizations are mindful about diversity, the opinion of most black people I meet is that 'veganism is a white privilege thing.' Thinking back to my childhood, there was no choice in what we ate; if it was put on the plate and placed in front of you, then that's what you had to eat. Acceptance of and gratitude for food were ingrained from an early age.

If I'm honest, sometimes I encounter what I feel are excuses. I understand, but I recognize a sad irony too. Why can't we just open our eyes and see that animals are enslaved as our ancestors once were. We have no right of ownership, and if anyone is capable of empathizing with animals as the victims of exploitation and greed, we should be. On the flip side, there's the reality of the world we live in today, a world in which we're still fighting against discrimination and prejudice, and

I guess it's difficult for people to put the welfare of animals before that of their own. In a perfect world, we'd all live by the golden rule: 'Treat all creatures as you wish to be treated.' What a wonderful world that would be.

Super-natural eating

Whatever the meat industry might like us to think, a plant-based diet shouldn't be considered eccentric. It's perfectly natural when you stop to think about it. Consider the original source of every vitamin and nutrient you consume as an omnivore. Is the original source of the nutrient the animal? Of course not! Protein, iron, potassium, calcium, all the B vitamins we get from animal products, their original source is the earth. We take the majority of our world's grains: the soy, wheat, corn and oats, and we feed these grains to billions of livestock. We only get the nutrients we require because the animals have eaten these plants. This seems like a colossal waste of effort and energy. When we eat animals and animal products, what we're doing is filtering our nutrients through the dead bodies of various animals. It doesn't make sense when you think of it this way.

Most of us have a limited understanding of nutrition, and limited time, patience or self-discipline when it comes to choosing what to eat. Set this in an environment where newspapers shout about the benefits or dangers of a different diet each week: 'Count calories', 'Don't count calories', 'Eat like a caveman',' 'Fast twice a week', 'Carbs make you fat', etc. Throw in a nod to the deep emotional associations we have with particular foods, and it's easy to see why taking an informed, dispassionate approach to eating is far easier said than done. Enter this book and my diet plan, which is designed to give your body what it needs: the macronutrients, in the right proportions to thrive.

More and more people are discovering the truth: food is medicine and medicine food. Through my network from my plant-based nutrition course, I'm finding more and more people who are curing themselves of their health conditions using nutrition. Their medical practitioner will prescribe pills for high blood pressure, pills for high cholesterol, pills for this, pills for that, and people may go on for years taking all these pills and managing the side effects. However, the medicines often mask or compensate for symptoms that are the result of poor lifestyle choices. Symptoms that could be more cheaply, simply and effectively relieved by changes to diet and lifestyle. When a lucky few of these people take matters into their own hands, switch to a plant-based diet and up their exercise, the results are often life-altering. No wonder such dramatic, natural improvements turn people into evangelical advocates of veganism and the gym.

Once you've spent a few weeks following my 12-week training programme and eating vegan, using the recipes in Chapters 7 and 8 as inspiration, I hope that you'll be feeling equally positive, ready to shout from the rooftops about the benefits of your new plant-based lifestyle.

Chapter 1

More Than Just
Fruit and Veg

Whether it's flexitarian, vegetarian, vegan or raw, there are a mind-scrambling variety of different ways to do it, and a range of labels from which to choose, for those wanting to reduce or eliminate animal products. Delicious vegan options are springing up on menus everywhere from high-street bakeries to fine dining restaurants. I for one am overjoyed that unchecked meat consumption seems to have had its day and enthusiastically welcome any label or initiative that helps us embark on a more conscious, plant-based lifestyle.

Different types of diet

Here's a quick lowdown on the different types of meat-reducing, veggie and vegan diets to choose from.

Meat-lite

Aside from traditional eat-everything carnivores and omnivores, a growing number of people are adopting a range of meat-reducing approaches to eating. This might begin with a commitment to meat-free Mondays, or Veganuary and go from there.

Flexitarian

This is a plant-based or vegetarian diet with the occasional serving of meat. Flexitarians do their best to limit meat intake as much as possible, and it works well for families who have previously relied on eating meat and dairy products. When you decide to stop basing every meal around meat, you begin to explore the broad range of alternative options available. This is a great place to start. Many of my clients come to me as meat-reducing flexitarians before deciding to go the whole way.

Pollotarian

Those who follow this type of diet don't consume red meat, fish or seafood. The only meat eaten is poultry and fowl. Chicken is our favourite meat in the UK, with poultry consumption overtaking beef for the first time ever in 2017. I used to LOVE chicken: the crispy skin and aroma of a roast – there really isn't anything like it. I know from what my clients tell me that most people believe that 'white' meat is less fatty and better for us.

They are shocked when I tell them that this is open to debate. We'll look at the science on the health impact of particular meats in Chapter 3.

Pescatarian

Those who follow a pescatarian diet don't eat meat, only fish, seafood and dairy. From a nutritional point of view, wanting to maintain a healthy intake of omega-3, this may seem appealing. However, once you begin to look into the realities of plastic pollution and heavy antibiotic and antifungal use in the fishing and fish-farming industries, you may change your mind.

Vegetarian

Vegetarianism is currently more popular than veganism, and some people might find it easier to be vegetarian, particularly those who have previously eaten a lot of meat and dairy. There are numerous studies showing that vegetarianism is beneficial to health.

- **Lacto-ovo vegetarian:** those who eat a lacto-ovo vegetarian diet don't consume red meat, white meat, fish or poultry. They do consume dairy and egg products. This is the most popular vegetarian type and is unquestionably more straightforward than a vegan diet. Those who are vegetarians will already have a food-carbon footprint almost half that of the average meat-eater (*see p.68*). Research has found that those who were already veggie before trying veganism are more likely to stick with it, so vegetarianism is a halfway house for those who are vegan-curious, but not sure if they want to go the whole way. It works well as a stepping-stone on the way to full veganism.

- **Ovo vegetarian:** this type of diet is meat- and dairy-free but includes eggs. I fully understand that eggs are one of the toughest things to give up and tend to be the food new clients miss most. Eggs are in so many things: they're a quick and easy solution for breakfast and lunch and are so useful in cakes and in cooking generally. While I'd love to say scrambled tofu is just as good, it would be a lie. However, with a bit of know-how, there are great cake recipes and breakfast options for vegans out there. I'll share a couple of them with you in Chapter 7.

Relaxed vegan

This kind of vegan isn't too concerned about the provenance and quality of food and eats a mixture of processed vegan foods alongside their vegetables. Many vegans who are new to the lifestyle, or particularly time-pressed (or feeding a family), fall into this camp.

Raw vegan

Raw vegans don't eat any processed foods, or any other food altered from its natural state. They believe that eating uncooked food provides living enzymes and proper nutrition, although the science behind this is open to debate. Raw vegans avoid any food cooked at a temperature above 48°C (118.5°F) as they believe cooking above this temperature results in the loss of a significant amount of nutritional value, rendering the food in question harmful to the body.

Plant-based whole food

A 'whole foods', plant-based diet encourages eating fruits and vegetables, and plenty of them. This diet includes lots of whole grains and means avoiding animal products, including all meats, fish, eggs, dairy and other foods such as honey. This is the approach I advocate working towards, and the meal plans and recipes in this book will help you to transition to this type of diet. I promise you won't regret it, and it's easier than you might think once you have the right support and advice.

You'll be in good company too, as more and more of us are recognizing the benefits of the vegan lifestyle. In the UK, 3.5 million people now identify as vegan. It's a figure that's jumped sharply from 2016, and the number is expected to keep rising as awareness grows around the environmental impact of consuming animal products.

Invest in your health

Here's a sign of the times: I have a good friend in the fire service who I played football with as a child. We've known each other for over 22 years. Lee is honestly the last person I'd ever expect to contemplate veganism, let alone give it a try. I'd even go as far as calling him anti-vegan. I've had various attempted debates with him in the past. I say attempted because I'd always listen to the point he was trying to make, but he didn't want to listen to anything I had to say. His mind was set, and there was no openness to change, but then, the unthinkable happened. I heard on the grapevine that he'd had an overnight change of heart and decided to switch to a vegan diet. I had to find out if it was true, and if it was, I was curious to know what the cause was. After all, I figured that if he could change, anyone could.

I reconnected with him and asked why the transition and his reason was simple: he'd read up on it. The information out there about the detrimental effect of eating meat and dairy products on our health is persuasive. He'd spent some time researching it and now wanted to change his diet radically. He has been happy with the results. A year on, and he's in the best condition of his life as well as being the healthiest and fittest he's ever been. Just like most of us who transition to a vegan lifestyle, the 'why factor' is quick to expand. Once you open the door to thinking more consciously about what you eat, awareness grows alongside increased empathy and compassion.

My friend is far from alone in his sudden shift in thinking. Countless people message me on social media every day, asking how it's done and questions such as, 'What exactly do you eat? How do you maintain a fit, muscular and athletic physique on a plant-based diet? Where do I get my protein from? They tell me they want to make the change but just don't know how best to do it. This book is my attempt to help people like Lee, who want to give this radical new lifestyle the best chance of success and sticking power.

We are investing in our health because we understand that we have to. Our health won't 'take care of itself'. The growing obesity epidemic and rise in chronic conditions from type 2 diabetes to auto-immune diseases means that more of us than ever are looking into lifestyle changes that can improve our health and longevity. Coupled with this, the anxiety of living in a rocky economic climate, with jobs less stable than ever, has led to a desire to take control of the areas of our lives where we can. Our exercise and dietary habits are an obvious place to start. Finally, technology and its distractions often mean we're always 'on' but have little time to think deeply about how we want to live. In reaction to all of this, people have begun to look within themselves, and start listening more to what works for their body. There's a movement away from blind consumerism to more conscious choices.

It makes a lot of sense, in this context that veganism is becoming more mainstream. Veganuary, which had its biggest year to date in 2019, is so inspiring. Even if those who sign up go back to eating an omnivorous diet afterwards, the impact that one meat- and dairy-free month has on the environment fills people with hope. And once people have dipped their toe in the water, I hope they'll have learned a range of tasty vegan meal options that they'll return to. Some of them will be inspired to keep eating vegan after January, too.

Making the switch

The challenge with going from zero to 60, though, even for a month, is that it's a tough adjustment. That's why this book will show you how to make the switch day by day: reducing your intake of animal products if you decide a gradual transition is the most likely to work for you. In this way, you'll start by replacing familiar animal-produce staples with pre-prepared vegan alternatives, rather than putting yourself under pressure to switch to a whole food, everything-from-scratch, vegan diet on day one. I've seen too many fledgling vegans fall into this trap and fail before. It's partly why I set up my coaching business, The Fit Vegan, where I move in with clients who are making the switch to veganism. It really helps to have someone with you; to show you what to cook and how to avoid falling off the bandwagon.

If, before deciding to go vegan, the client has tended to rely on processed foods and fish- or meat-and-two-veg-style dinners, I advise them to avoid romanticizing the likelihood of whipping up exotic and elaborate Ottolenghi salads or vegan curries made with a paste made from scratch every night. I recommend being realistic and thinking about what will give them the best chance of success. So that goes for you, too.

Of course, this book will help you decide how best to set about making the change, with meal plans, recipes and shopping lists designed to support you. But before we get into the practicalities of what to eat and how to transition to plant-based eating, let's explore what it means to be vegan.

Motivations for change

I'm not facetious. Of course, I know there's a dictionary definition for vegan, but the motivations for choosing this lifestyle vary widely, and I think it's worth looking at all of them in turn. Here are the three most common:

Environmental

The leading scientists released their report on the 'planetary diet' earlier this year in *The Lancet*.[1] Their consensus? Switching to a mostly plant-based diet is the most dramatic way to reduce our carbon footprint, with researchers at the University of Oxford calculating switching to eating vegan reduces the average person's dietary footprint by up to 73 per cent.[2]

Compassionate

For ethical vegans, the welfare of animals is the primary motivator. A study last year by Global Data found that 50 per cent of vegans cited ethical reasons as their primary motivation when choosing to make the switch.[3-4] Ethical vegans question humans' right to kill and exploit animals for food and clothing. It is the reason most often cited by children for wanting to cut out animal products, too. Interestingly, a study by researchers at the University of Albany, USA, found that the more pets and the wider variety of pets that people had as they grew up, the more likely they were to be vegetarian or vegan as adults.[5] I notice in clients who have pets that the compassionate motivators for going vegan tend to be stronger.

Health

Modern life is exhausting, we're depleted by a work and lifestyle culture that demands a lot of us. Stress and anxiety are an almost universal daily experience for many people. But there's a shift happening, with more and more people prioritizing self-care and trying a range of practices – from mindfulness to dietary and exercise – to support their wellbeing. The popularity of veganism is part of this trend. Those who go plant-based for health reasons are picking up on the growing body of research suggesting that such diets significantly reduce the risk of chronic diseases, from obesity to type 2 diabetes. Books such as *The China Study* and *How Not to Die*, as well as vegan documentaries such as *Forks Over Knives*, focus on the staggering number of scientific studies that demonstrate links between chronic disease and the consumption of animal products. These links (to the development of conditions such as type 2 diabetes and heart disease, as well as cancer incidents), are incremental and well documented. We know that the more meat and dairy people eat, the higher their risk of developing a range of diseases. Sadly, the medical establishment has been slow to catch on to this research. As I mentioned previously, nutritional training for doctors is scant, and government guidelines on nutrition often lag behind the research, or (if we're more cynical about it) are diluted due to the lobbying power of the food industry.

Of course, it's a bit misleading to separate these three motivations as most of us are driven by a combination of all of them, and the unique cocktail will vary from day to day, too. A news report on the climate-change impact of the meat industry will tip us towards environmental motivation one day, while news of another family member or friend being diagnosed with cancer may sway us back to the health benefits of plant-based eating the next. Ultimately, it doesn't matter what motivates us, but it's important to understand your personal 'why' when it comes to maintaining motivation and resolve.

Compassion in action

I previously thought that vegan was just vegan: you either are or you're not. I also used to think vegans were weird. That was the old me, who didn't really have a clue. I'm now a firm believer that the type of vegan you are depends on the reasons you made the transition. I initially made the transition for ethical reasons. I care about animals and the environment, and I believe in equality for all living beings. But being an ethical vegan made my overnight transition to veganism a problematic start. I had an epiphany; I knew there was no going back. I couldn't cut down my meat consumption gradually because I couldn't bear the thought of eating it at all. I went from eating meat at any time of the day, not really caring about recycling, or my carbon footprint, to not wanting to harm a fly.

Once I started to look into the meat industry and think more about farming and animal slaughter, and the impact of the food I'd been eating (on the environment, my body and most of all, on animals) it was as if I was jolted awake. I had the passion and conviction I was doing the right thing, but the radical behavioural shift was SO HARD. I massively underestimated how deeply ingrained my eating habits were, and how tough it would be to adjust to a new way of cooking and eating. But I got through it, and I can share all the mistakes I made along the way to ensure you're better prepared and supported. The thing that kept me going was my conviction that I was doing the right thing, in a personal and moral sense.

This very passion is precisely what puts off some meat-eaters from even entertaining the idea of considering the benefits of a plant-based diet. I can understand the resistance. To be honest, I think I might have been a bit annoying when I first made the change because I wanted to scream it from the rooftops. My enthusiasm didn't go down well with everyone, and it caused more unproductive conflict than helpful discussion. It taught me only to share my experiences when asked, and to know that my personal choice isn't for everyone… no matter how great I think it is.

Even so, although it's not my job to judge other people for their lifestyle choices, or to preach, I do think there's real value in considering the ethical reasons for becoming vegan and being upfront about them to ourselves. Vegan philosophy promotes respect for life and compassion for all living beings by encouraging the active practice of *ahimsa*. This is an acronym with Sanskrit roots and means to cause no injury or do no harm by living by the following rules:

- Abstinence from animal products
- Harmlessness with reverence for life

- Integrity of thought, word and deed
- Mastery over oneself
- Service to humanity, nature and creation
- Advancement of understanding and truth

Ahimsa is also related to the notion that any violence has karmic consequences. This is why ethical vegans don't believe that animals are a resource to be exploited and don't eat any animal foods or their by-products, nor do they wear any animal skins (i.e. leather, fur, wool or silk).

For me, identifying as an ethical vegan represents strength. Having the courage of my convictions to stand up for what I believe to be right and just, to change my habits, and to go against the grain socially. Being vegan means being authentic and living in a way that's in tune with my core values. It also feels good knowing that, at the end of the day, no animals have suffered or been exploited to feed or clothe me. Ethical veganism is compassion in action. It's compassionate in the broadest sense of the word, encompassing compassion towards all other species and life forms with whom we share this planet. Ethical veganism is empathy: it enables us to see things from the Earth's, and other species', point of view. As humans, it's in our natures to be utterly egotistical. Choosing to put the lives of animals before my own pleasure has become a powerful antidote to this urge to please only myself, with no regard for the suffering that this might cause as collateral.

Ethical veganism is kindness, one of the greatest gifts that can both change and save a life; it's a manifestation of love. To love others as you love yourself. Just as we do, animals feel fear, love, happiness, pain, suffering and misery. Just like us, they have every desire to live and to be free. As I continue on my path and learn more, my personal definition of veganism expands. What was once a decision purely based on animal welfare has now become so much more.

Saying yes to ethical veganism

To sum it up, the designer leather jackets that used to have pride of place in my wardrobe have been given away. I no longer own leather shoes or silk pillowcases. Even cashmere jumpers and wool beanies are out. I won't take my daughter to the zoo, or a circus with animals, ever again. As soon as I began to think about where my food and clothes had come from, I found it profoundly upsetting that I'd felt no association with animals when I'd been wearing their skin. I'm so fascinated by how our minds have been conditioned from birth.

In light of this, it isn't surprising that changing our minds and our habits take time and patience. It feels like hard work to challenge the status quo, and our thought habits can be stubbornly rigid and resistant to disruption. I want to encourage you to say YES to:

- Creating filling, nutritious meals you enjoy

- Eating real food that gives you real energy

- Doing simple, speedy and effective workouts that'll get you fit, fast

- Making choices that fit with your authenticity

And NO to:

- Punishing diet regimes and faddish eating

- Buying expensive supplements and shakes

- Wasting hours on end in the gym

- Mindlessly following the crowd

Through this book, I'm hoping to help you do just that.

Chapter 2

No-Meat Muscle

So, let's tackle the biggest myth out there about veganism: it'll leave you weak, at risk of anaemia, lacking in energy and you'll struggle to build muscle. In fact, nothing could be further from the truth.

Protein, like the other macronutrients (carbohydrates and fats), is an essential part of a healthy diet. To build and repair muscle tissue, organs and bones, we undoubtedly need protein. But how much? Protein has become big business, with vested interests perhaps distorting our perception of how much we really need. The whey (milk-based) protein industry alone is worth $6.9 billion globally, which is predominantly a result of the bodybuilding industry. Supplement companies sponsor athletes and celebrities who promote their products, which in turn inspires their fans to purchase the product. This is the cycle that will likely lead to serious harm in the long term. Do a quick Google search, and you'll see how often ill-health and, sometimes, premature death affect bodybuilders. This is probably due to a combination of performance-enhancing drugs and diet-related health issues. So, my advice to anyone who is supplementing with protein is to say 'No' to whey protein and casein. These are both derived from cow's milk, and later in the book, I'll share with you why I believe dairy is scary and why we really should keep our distance. I'm on a mission to bust this protein myth, and my motivating factor is simply *your health*. I continue to go from strength to strength following a whole food plant-based diet.

The protein myth

I've heard this question so many times, often dressed up in different ways. At numerous gyms, bodybuilders have taken me aside and asked in a 'just between us' undertone, 'How do you really get your protein? Come on, tell me the truth.' And I continuously get DMs on social media along the same lines. With my clients too, the number-one excuse for falling off the vegan wagon is: 'But Ed, I really needed the protein.' More concerning is that a wide range of health professionals I've met and told about my passion for plant-based nutrition have repeated this age-old view back to me: 'It's tough to get enough protein as a vegan.'

Luckily for us, we'll always have a choice. What do you want to do? Simply take everyone's word for it or look further afield and make that informed decision based on credible advice on the nutrients you need when you're working out what to eat.

I've been eating a vegan diet for more than three years now. When I started, I believed I already had an excellent understanding of nutrition and how it affected the human body. It's something I've been interested in for a long time and, as a bodybuilder, I'd spent a lot of time researching. But since becoming vegan and adapting my diet, I've radically changed my perspective on nutrition. I discovered that I'd bought into a 'protein myth': I believed I needed far more protein than I really did to maintain and build muscle. I was getting 200–240g of animal protein daily as an omnivore, the ideal amount according to traditional bodybuilding knowledge, which recommends 1–1.5 grammes of protein per pound of body weight per day. But once I started to look beyond fitness magazines and bodybuilding blogs, searching for credible scientific evidence to back this up, I simply couldn't find any proof.

The evidence to support the amount of protein I was consuming was extremely flimsy. We know that the average Western diet delivers too much protein, which is why it's so unusual to hear about protein deficiency.[1–3] As I researched more and more about plant-based nutrition, I discovered the amount of protein humans need is a hotly debated topic. I've reduced my protein further in the past year after I came across a meta-analysis (a large study taking its results from several other studies) that measured the effect of protein supplementation in resistance training.[4] It showed optimal results could be achieved with a far lower protein intake than had previously been thought necessary. Protein, it turns out, has been seriously overhyped by the bodybuilding community.

When you're bodybuilding, the aim is to tear your muscle fibres (microtears), which the body will then repair using protein. You want to achieve an optimal amount of microtearing, and consuming sufficient protein to repair and grow the muscles is a necessity. I was shocked when I began to look into the numbers myself. As somebody who had trained consistently since my teens, through my 20s and into my 30s, I'm a former meathead who has often supplemented my meat and egg-based meals with extra protein in the form of whey powders and supplements.

I couldn't believe I'd been consuming so much unnecessary animal protein under the misguided belief that I needed it to gain and retain muscle. My fridge had been packed with pints of milk, and I'd sometimes guzzle most of a bottle at breakfast, and eat chicken, minced beef and veg from my plastic Tupperware containers. I didn't even like milk, I never have. I only drank it because I was told it would make me big and strong and give me healthy bones. My cupboards were full of huge plastic tubs of whey protein powders, and various boxes of protein bars that I considered 'healthy snacks'. Sure, I noticed a benefit from eating these, but only (I understand in retrospect), because they were providing me with nutrients I should have had in my diet already in the form of healthy food.

I'd been a sucker for the persuasive marketing budgets of the protein powders and supplements companies. This smart marketing led me up the garden path, as it has many others. I can't bear to think about the amount of money I wasted on unnecessary fake food.

Despite the fact I realized I'd been mistaken about protein, after years of consuming lots of it, drastically reducing my intake felt a bit scary. I was worried I'd lose strength. But as I got used to it, and kept on training, increasing the intensity of my exercise regime and reducing my protein intake, I continued to make progress. The proof was in the pudding for me.

I now know that the amount of protein I require for optimum health is 5–10 per cent of my total calories per day. This is a tiny amount in comparison to the other macronutrients (carbohydrates and fat). It should now be clear to see that as long as you're consuming enough calories daily, you'd struggle to suffer from a protein deficiency even if you tried.

Calculating your daily fuel

So how should you go about calculating how much protein you need to fuel your lifestyle? The EAR is the estimated average daily requirement (for the population). It's the scale used by the experts at Cornell and the plant-based nutrition course I'm studying. It was formerly known as the minimum daily requirement, but considering emerging research, some are using it as a guideline for optimal nutrition. The EAR suggests 0.5–0.6g protein per 1kg of body weight per day is the requirement, considerably less than the bodybuilding figure I used to go by!

First up, let's dispel the idea that animal products are essential for protein. What if I told you that a woman who weighs 60kg needs only 30–45g of protein per day. And if she were to eat the following meals and snacks, she'd be getting more than she needs, and plenty to support an intensive training regime:

Breakfast (10.5g protein): porridge made with soy milk (9g protein) and 50g stewed dried apricots (1.5g protein)

Snack (1.8g protein): 150g punnet raspberries (1.8g protein)

Lunch (12.5g protein): bowl of lentil soup (8g protein), with half an avocado (1.5g protein) on a slice of whole wheat toast (3g protein)

Snack (6g protein): 1 serving of almonds (6g protein)

Dinner (14g protein): 50g falafel (6.5g protein) with 15g of hummus (0.75g protein), 75g quinoa served with finely chopped beef tomato, a drizzle of olive oil and parsley (7.5g protein), 190g broccoli (2.5g protein)

Men don't require much more than this – just work it out according to your body weight (your weight in kilogrammes × 0.5 is the number of grammes of protein you need per day).

Vegan muscle

Now, I don't go in for any of the gels, shakes or isotonic drinks, and I get my protein from lentils, tofu, quinoa, buckwheat, tempeh and plenty of veg on the side. I occasionally use a combination of brown rice and pea protein because they have a high amino-acid profile. The more essential amino acids, the better! Hard data acts as proof that I'm stronger than ever on a plant-based diet eating only real food I've prepared myself. Since I've gone vegan, my pound-for-pound strength has increased, and I feel more energized and stronger than I previously did eating meat and dairy products. I'm a bit of a fitness geek, so I've felt motivated and fascinated by recording the details of the physical and mental changes I've noticed and measured since going vegan. I've shared my journey on Instagram, and the response has been really inspiring.

The biggest surprise has been the unexpected fitness benefits I've experienced. Surprising because my focus at the beginning was on maintenance rather than improvement. But the gains have been significant. My endurance has increased considerably since I've stopped eating animal products. Long-distance running used to KILL me, but now I can keep on going, comfortably, for at least 15 miles. In the past, I'd have proclaimed I simply didn't have the physique for endurance exercise: power and strength were my forte. But now I can see that many of the assumptions I made about my body and my fitness were based on my response to an unhealthy diet high in animal products that left me feeling sluggish and heavy.

As I always say, the proof is in the pudding. Using my new Tanita scale recommended by a good friend, I put plant-based eating to the test and followed my weightlifting programme to see how I'd fare. It's essential not just to look at weight as this is only a small piece of the puzzle. What is much more of a useful measure of physical condition is body composition. The table opposite demonstrates my results after nine weeks of vigorous training consuming less than half the amount of protein than I did previously.

As you can see, my exercise regime and a balanced plant-based diet in which I consumed a daily surplus of 500 calories, resulted in me losing body fat and gaining muscle mass simultaneously (this is where calorie counting is essential). If you just want to be fit and healthy, train hard and eat well. However, if you're aiming for specific goals regarding weight and body composition, you'll get there so much more quickly if you're SMART about it I'll talk more about SMART goals later in the book (see pp.84–85).

Body composition	Week 1	Week 2	Week 3	Week 4	Week 5	Week 6	Week 7	Week 8	Week 9
Weight (kg)	90.2	90.8	91.4	92.1	92.6	93.2	93.8	94.8	95
BMI	30.7	30.6	30.7	29.7	29.5	28.1	27.9	27.5	26
Body fat %	17.5	16.5	15.2	15.1	14.8	14.1	13.3	12.5	11
Muscle mass (kg)	72.5	73.7	73.9	74.8	75.3	75.3	76.1	80	80.2
Physique rating	6	6	6	6	6	6	6	9	9
Bone mass (kg)	3.7	3.7	3.7	3.8	3.8	3.9	3.9	4.0	4.0
Visceral fat	8.5	8.0	7.5	7.5	6.5	6.0	6.0	5.5	5
BMR	2,204	2,295	2,321	2,370	2,424	2,483	2,501	2,559	2,670
Metabolic age	25	25	24	23	21	21	20	19	19
Total body water %	56.5	58.5	59	59.5	59.5	60	61.5	61.5	62

My training plan*

* These results were achieved with a daily surplus of 500kcal, which should support a weight increase of around 0.5kg (about a 1lb) a week in most people, but results depend on body type. If you don't build muscle quickly, a portion of that weight will inevitably be stored as fat.

As you can see from the table, following a plant-based diet and hypertrophy training (for growth in muscle mass), my body composition improved week by week, as did my strength. In case any of the terms are new to you, here follows a glossary of calculations:

Weight: total weight or mass of your body.

BMI: standard ratio of weight to height, used as a general indication of health for the average population.

Body fat percentage: proportion of fat to total body weight. Body fat is essential for cushioning joints and protecting your internal organs, and also helps to maintain body temperature.

Muscle mass: predicted weight of muscle in the body – including skeletal muscle, smooth muscle and the heart.

Physique rating: assessment of muscle and body-fat levels that rates its results as one of nine body types: one being the highest body fat and lowest muscle mass; nine being the lowest body fat and highest muscle mass.

Bone mass: predicted weight of bone mineral in the body.

Visceral fat: this is located deep in the core abdominal area that surrounds and protects the vital organs. It is often the result of overindulgence and referred to as 'stubborn fat'.

BMR: basal metabolic rate is the minimum daily amount of energy the body requires when at rest (including when asleep) to function effectively. My BMR increased week by week, meaning I'd be burning more calories at rest, helping me to reduce body fat. I used my BMR as a minimum baseline for my diet programme.

Metabolic age: comparison of your BMR to an average for your age group.

Total body water: total amount of fluid in the body expressed as a percentage of your total weight.

Lean, keen and OD-ing on protein

As anyone who has spent a fair bit of time hanging around at the gym will tell you, overconsumption of animal protein and dairy-based powders can result in some unpleasant side effects. These range from the antisocial (noxious flatulence: meat contains high levels of sulphur which makes wind smellier), the uncomfortable (chronic constipation is typical in weightlifters, thanks to protein overload) and the dangerous (kidney and liver damage can result from prolonged overconsumption). I recently heard of a bodybuilder at a friend's gym who was rushed to hospital following kidney failure as a consequence of years' worth of overdoing the protein. A cautionary tale we should all pay attention to.

Before I discovered the benefits of a plant-based diet, I used to down whey protein (milk-based) drinks almost every day.

A typical day might include six eggs, salmon and avocado for breakfast, chicken and rice for lunch and a similar dinner, occasionally swapping the chicken out for tilapia (fish). I aimed for 1–1.5g of protein per 0.5kg (1lb) of bodyweight a day, which is twice what I eat now. It was far more than I needed. Over time, my digestion slowed and (apologies for the overshare, but I promise it's relevant), I got constipated on a few occasions. I only put two and two together and realized protein was the culprit when I reduced my protein consumption and upped my fruit and veg, and finally found usual service was restored to my bowels. Hallelujah! It was a revelation, and I couldn't believe I hadn't worked it out sooner.

A life-changing decision

Despite feeling the benefits within days of going vegan, clear evidence that my body worked better on a plant-based diet, I still had a voice in my head whispering that really, I needed meat to maintain muscle mass, and I came close to wavering in the first few weeks. I just couldn't equate veganism with fitness and strength. I had images of waifish yogis and 'clean eating' models in my mind. When I look back now, I'm actually amazed that I ignored all that prejudice and went for it anyway. It felt like a real leap of faith going plant-based, which I did overnight.

On my first day as a vegan, I felt great! Even before breakfast, I was overcome with a sense of joy. Simply knowing that I was no longer contributing to the pain and suffering of animals lifted my spirit. Eggs and salmon were now a thing of the past, but oats, bananas, nuts and seeds, along with unsweetened almond milk gave me everything I needed and more to kickstart my day.

Soon after the transition, I began to follow a cardio-based exercise routine. Running and endurance had always been my fitness nemesis. The first time I took to the roads was when I noticed the power that plant-based nutrition had on me. A slow 3-mile jog turned into a quick 3-mile run. Just like that.

I didn't really investigate plant-based nutrition for many months following my transition. I remained eating as always, minus the animal products. So, for example, I was eating sweet potatoes or quinoa, with an array of vegetables. Half my plate would always be filled with salad, including plenty of spinach. I felt great. Lighter, happier and a lot more agile.

Why a plant-based diet supports a healthy body

If you're not yet fully convinced about taking the plunge, I'd like to share eight reasons why I believe plant-based diets are the best way to support a fit, healthy, athletic body:

#1 Vegans are NO MORE LIKELY to be anaemic than meat-eaters

Iron is essential for energy, and a deficiency will leave you feeling weak and tired: not ideal if exercise is important to you. You've probably heard that veggies and vegans are more likely to be deficient in iron. For anyone who cares about fitness, this is likely to be a significant concern. But a closer look at the evidence shows there's nothing much to back up this pervasive belief. Yep, you heard that right. A 1994 study found that iron deficiency anaemia was no higher in those eating a vegan diet.[5] A subsequent wide-ranging study more recently in 2009 by the American Dietetic Association (not generally known for their progressive stance on avoiding animal products), with data drawn from a range of studies, states that: 'Incidence of iron-deficiency anaemia among vegetarians is similar to that of nonvegetarians.'[6]

So why are veggies and vegans no more likely to be anaemic if meat offers a far more 'bio-available' source of iron than plant-based sources? It's partly because dairy decreases iron absorption by up to 50 per cent. And partially because vegans naturally eat more vitamin C-rich foods that significantly increase iron absorption. Vegetarians also eat more iron overall than most meat-eaters, although the iron in meat is the more readily absorbed heme type. Too much heme iron can lead to constipation, stomach pain and nausea, and excessive supplementation has been found to lead to an elevated risk of liver and bowel cancer as well as type 2 diabetes.[7] Having said all that, if you're worried about your iron levels, cutting down on caffeine, which interferes with iron absorption, and drinking a glass of OJ with your meal will boost your iron absorption.

#2 Vegans don't stink out the gym

I've been tempted to share this wisdom more than once when I've been training downwind of a whey enthusiast! Is there anything worse than being that person on the weights bench or yoga mat who emits a noisy and noxious cloud of methane? Despite the anti-bean propaganda, milk and dairy products are one of the leading causes of excess windiness, mainly due to the surprising number of people who are lactose intolerant. If you're of East, Central and Southern Asian origin, or African or Afro-Caribbean heritage, you're far more likely to suffer from this affliction than most Caucasians. Some studies put lactose intolerance at around 90 per cent for some populations, so it might be worth investigating your risk.[8]

We know that the worst-smelling farts come from high-sulphur foods, such as meat and eggs, but what about the bean thing? Several studies have measured whether upping consumption of legumes leads to a matching increase in incidence and quantity of wind. Research reveals a mixed picture, with minor and temporary increases in flatulence appearing to fade after a few weeks. Researchers concluded the windy reputation of beans had been exaggerated.[9] Either way, a low-level increase (and a temporary one, at that), is a small price to pay for the massive range of benefits that come from eating legumes, and even if they cause a bit of wind, at least it won't smell anything like meat-loving Mike's.

#3 Vegetables count as 'performance-enhancing' substances

To take one incredible example, beetroot has been shown to enhance performance in endurance cycling to the extent that athletes drinking nitrate-rich beetroot juice before a long ride saw an astonishing increase in their oxygen efficiency and endurance.[10] The benefit exceeded improvements in oxygen uptake shown in previous studies focusing on sprint training, endurance training and even hyperoxia (in which athletes wear a mask to breathe a higher percentage of oxygen while exercising). In a 2009 study, cyclists were able to work at the same intensity with 19 per cent less oxygen uptake than a placebo group. In the same study, those who had drunk the beetroot juice took 90 seconds longer to reach exhaustion than the non-beetroot group.[11] Imagine that, the Tour de France team cool bags filled with beetroot juice in unmarked vials. Just a single shot of beetroot juice has been found to allow free-divers to hold their breath for half-a-minute longer than usual, and similar benefits have been observed in runners, too. Eating beetroot, a couple of hours before training, should give you a boost. Why not try it: grate raw beetroot into a sandwich, salad or slaw, or cook it with tomatoes, vegetable stock and a little garlic to make a delicious, and nutritious 'red soup'.

#4 Legumes tick the 'high-quality' protein box

Until recently, the dietary assessment of protein quality was based on the impact of different foods on rats. This led to the undervaluing of the quality of protein from legumes. This is one of the reasons that so many misunderstandings have arisen about the capacity of vegan diets to deliver enough protein. Now, the WHO (World Health Organization) has adopted an alternative way to measure protein efficiency, correcting for human digestibility. The protein scores of beans, when measured in this new way, are better.[12] Soybeans, in particular, score extremely highly on the revised scale.[13]

#5 Vegan diets strike the perfect ratio

Even the most mainstream omnivorous diet advice recommends eating a high ratio of vegetables and complex carbohydrates to protein. More cutting edge diets that aren't limited by association with major food producers, such as Michael Pollan's,[14] advocate a 'mostly' plant-based approach. By choosing a vegan diet, you take the hard work out of the calculations as you'll already be drawing your calories from plants. Vegans and vegetarians eat far fewer calories than omnivores, on average, which has been shown to improve metabolism and reduce central obesity, both of which will help to balance the hormones leptin and ghrelin that regulate appetite.

#6 Vegan muscles bounce back faster

As any athlete knows, recovery between training sessions is essential. Adequate recovery enhances performance and endurance and allows the body to repair itself. 'No pain, no gain' has more than a grain of truth in it – the only way to build muscle is to overload your muscles progressively by challenging them to exhaustion. Endless reps with light weights, for example, are a real waste of time. Having said that, there's no need to suffer more than you need to, and a vegan diet will help you to bounce back from a workout more quickly.

I've experienced the difference this makes first-hand. I used to suffer really badly with DOMS (delayed onset muscle soreness), pain resulting from the microtears in my muscles 12–72 hours after training. When I was eating a meat-based diet, it would sometimes take three days for the soreness to subside after an intense workout. At its worst, DOMS can disrupt training and throw the best-laid plans out of the window. It feels terrible, too. From a physiological point of view, the pain is a result of inflammation, the body's response to the oxidative damage of exercise. Foods that raise muscle-glycogen levels are what the body needs to repair the damage. These are found in carbohydrates, and plant-based carbs and whole grains are the best sources. Making sure you have enough protein is important too, so keep an eye on your intake. Now, I allow myself plenty of rest, but I recover from DOMS far more quickly and experience it less. Perhaps it's because my diet is packed with anti-inflammatory plant nutrients? This seems a likely explanation.

#7 Vegans have more stamina

The image of meat is one of strength. We associate it with satiation and sustenance, and it taps into the hunter-gatherer idea of feasting on sustaining proteins. But what if this is little more than a macho nostalgic fantasy? In a famous study at Yale way back in 1907, even sedentary vegetarians had greater stamina than meat-eaters who exercised – with sedentary meat-eaters coming off worst of all in the tests.[15-17]

Think about some of the world's most muscular mammals – gorillas and elephants are two that spring to mind, although there are many more – that are vegan. Just saying.

#8 Vegans are less likely to play the toxic credit-debit game

A trap that many people fall into is adopting the mindset of training hard during the week and treating themselves at the weekend. On the surface, the odds seem to be stacked in your favour; it looks balanced as there are five days in the week and two days at the weekend. But take a closer look and do some quick maths, and you'll realize that weekends count for 104 days out of 365. Now, that's what I'd not only call counterproductive but also working against your goals. In addition to the weekends, you also have birthday celebrations, weddings, holidays, festive seasons like Christmas and Thanksgiving, and let's not forget the times you just feel like pigging out.

Can you see how quickly that 104 becomes most of the year? It's essential to stay focused and keep your eye on the goal. Don't think you can 'get away' with ordering that stuffed-crust pepperoni pizza because you just did a circuit session, or reaching for a second serving of ice cream after a long training run. Foods that are high in fat, salt and protein are moreish and addictive, and when you combine this with a credit–debit mindset, which so many of us fall into, you can end up undoing so much of your excellent work by making poor food choices. Limiting the poor food choices available to you as you do when you go vegan might be a crude way to restrict temptation, but it's an effective one, and what's more, a plant-based diet will retrain your palate to crave healthier foods.

Chapter 3

Healthy Choices

N ext, I'm going to state something you think might be obvious: a whole food vegan diet is really, really good for you. Eating a whole food vegan diet means you'll eat more portions of fruit and veg than the average omnivore. By following the meal plans in this book, you'll get to 7–10 portions of fruit and veg per day. In the course of my research into veganism, I learned that those who eat seven or more portions of fruit and veg a day have a 33 per cent reduced risk of premature death.[1] Similarly, a meta-analysis of 95 studies by researchers at Imperial College London in 2017, which was based on the dietary habits of two million people around the world, found that the maximum preventative health benefit was seen in people eating 10 or more portions of fruit and veg per day.[2] Data from the study included 43,000 cases of heart disease, 47,000 cases of stroke, 81,000 cases of cardiovascular disease, 112,000 cancer cases and 94,000 deaths, and it makes a strong case that diets high in plant-based foods are the healthiest.

Of course, not all of those eating the 10 portions a day were vegetarian or vegan, but when you're eating a plant-based diet, it's certainly easier to hit that magic number! That isn't to say that unhealthy vegans don't exist. But before we get into the specifics of how to eat a balanced vegan diet, let's take a look at the average Western diet. The kind I ate until five years ago.

The 'not so perfect' human diet

Most of us are omnivores while 2–4 per cent of the UK population identify as vegetarian or vegan (although 21 per cent describe themselves as 'meat reducers': eating less meat than they did before).[3] I've noticed more and more of my friends cutting back on their meat consumption recently, which is an encouraging sign that times are changing. Vegans, although rapidly growing in number, still represent a minority.

For those wanting to weigh up the impact of switching from an omnivorous to a vegan diet, the sheer volume of conflicting information can make it seem like a daunting, perhaps even impossible, task. It creates a climate of confusion, and I know from what my clients tell me, it can feel difficult to know which research to trust. Ideas about the health and wholesomeness of meat and dairy are deeply embedded in our thinking. As a child, I remember being told that eggs were a 'perfect', healthy food and that I needed to drink up my school milk to build strong bones. Of course, if I wanted to have strong muscles, lean meats were the key thing to include in my diet. Sure, too much saturated fat was bad news, so limiting the bacon was to be recommended. But meats and dairy were good enough for our caveman ancestors, right? What I forgot, though, is that for caveman ancestors, meat was an occasional treat. People mainly subsisted on roots and berries. And just as they weren't eating bagels, biscuits or crisps, they weren't eating sausages, either, or having steak for dinner every day.

When I started to investigate the impact that my massive meat and egg consumption was likely to be having on my body, I became geekily absorbed in the evidence. I discovered that there's a growing body of evidence to show that animal products (particularly those produced in the way they tend to be now, on substantial industrial farms, consumed in large quantities, every day), can be bad news for our health.

As I read more and more about the benefits of a healthy vegan diet, I discovered that the Academy of Nutrition and Dietetics in the USA has stated that vegans boast lower overall cancer rates, lower rates of ischaemic heart disease and type 2 diabetes, lower blood cholesterol and blood pressure levels, as well as lower rates of hypertension.[4]

Aside from reading nutrition features in health and fitness magazines or getting tips from the net and other guys in the gym, I hadn't delved too deeply into the science until that point. I was fit, I felt good, looked healthy, and I enjoyed my meat- and dairy-heavy diet, so I hadn't seen the need. Now, I shudder to think of how oblivious and disinterested I was about the food I was putting into my body. I didn't really give it a second thought.

Flash forward three years, where I've devoted myself to discovering as much as I can about healthy eating, and I'm a passionate believer that we all need more information to make informed decisions about our food choices. I believe that for years I put my life at risk with my overconsumption of meat and dairy products. Nothing upsets me more than the memory of seeing my mum deteriorate as we, her family, unknowingly sat back and continued to watch her consume the diet that may have contributed to the illness in the first instance. My mother was far from exceptional in her diagnosis as cancer, heart disease and strokes are the leading causes of death in the world we live in today.

Now that there's more evidence than ever to link the foods we eat to these major diseases, why wouldn't we want to change our habits for the sake of our health? We know now that diet can have a preventative impact on disease risk. Some studies show that in certain cancers, such as early-stage prostate cancer, the disease may even be reversed by switching to a whole food, plant-based diet,[5] which is why perhaps a plant-based diet may have had an effect on Malaika's precancerous cells. When my father was diagnosed with prostate cancer last year, I immediately put together a meal plan for him. It wasn't early-stage prostate cancer but had spread to his pelvis and breastbone. He contemplated chemotherapy for all of two seconds before opting out. Eating a plant-based diet is something he'd have laughed at before his diagnosis. Dad still has cancer but now he takes two medications daily instead of five, says he feels better than ever and seems to be in great shape and high spirits. With each test taken, there are minor improvements. His doctor often tells him, 'Thomas, whatever you're doing, you just keep on doing it.' I simply call it plant power.

Knowing that heart disease could, for many, be prevented and even reversed with nutrition alone should be something we're taught in school.[6-7] I certainly wish I'd been made aware of the power of food to prevent illness. Another example that jumped at me from the research I uncovered was about stroke, another leading cause of death and disability in the UK. My uncle died of a stroke in 2011, so it's a subject close to my heart. Numerous studies have shown that fruit and veg are protective against ischaemic strokes (the type caused by blood clots).

A real wakeup-call for me came when I read the headlines about the WHO report in 2015, saying: 'Regular consumption of processed meat ranked alongside smoking as a major cause of cancer.'[8] Bearing in mind that I've lost several family members and friends to cancer, I felt obliged to double-check it. The research explicitly related to rectal/colon cancer. At this point, I was still eating a meat-heavy diet, and I stopped to count the number of portions of processed meat I'd eat in an average week. Granted, it was only three or so servings, but consuming something I knew was detrimental to my health made no sense to me. I wouldn't smoke a cigarette, so why would I eat processed meat? I thought about my mother cooking up corned-beef stews in our many times of hardship, my two aunts and the processed meats they would sometimes eat. Uncle Fred's favourite dish, carbonara. I couldn't help but wonder whether the diet was part of the reason why so many of my family members had become cancer statistics.

Then there were the links to type 2 diabetes. I always believed this developed as a result of a high-sugar diet. Admittedly, this is true, but the more I read, the more I learned about the possible links between diabetes and the high consumption of animal products. I sifted through the studies and was reminded of so many memories of visiting extended family in the USA, with buffet tables laden with ham, fried chicken and creamy, mayo-heavy sauces. There would always be several people with type 2 diabetes there, suffering the discomfort and life-limiting consequences of this 'lifestyle' disease, while the rest of us loaded our plates with unhealthy food. Something about this felt so wrong.

Five good health reasons to make the switch

Here are some exciting discoveries I've made in my research about the physical impact of the sort of diet I used to eat, one based around meat and animal-product consumption. I hope it provides you with some extra information and context when you're making choices about how to improve your own diet.

#1 The WHO says there's no 'safe' amount of processed meat

I used to eat bacon sandwiches at least a couple times a week. I knew they weren't really good for me, but I figured that I did lots of fitness training and was generally healthy, so how bad could they really be? Turns out they may have been doing me more damage than I thought. We now know that all processed meats (i.e. bacon, sausages, ham, chicken nuggets) are harmful to our health. When I stumbled across the WHO report categorizing meats including bacon, frankfurters and ham, as group 1 carcinogens (meaning they're known to cause cancer), I wanted to understand more. I learned that each 50g portion (equivalent to 1.5–2 deli slices of ham) eaten per day increased my risk of digestive cancer by 18 per cent. Once I started Googling, I found another study linked even moderate processed-meat consumption (equivalent to less than a rasher of bacon a day) to a 21 per cent increased risk of breast cancer.[9] In short, the WHO summed it up by saying there's no 'safe' minimum amount of processed meat we can eat.[10]

What about unprocessed red meat, I wondered? I'd long considered a lean steak and salad as a super-healthy food full of high-quality protein. I was shocked to discover that for every portion of red meat we eat per day, our risk of premature death increases by 13 per cent.[11] And in a large study in 2017 looking at the diets of over 500,000 men and women aged 50–71 over 16 years, those who ate the most red meat experienced a 26 per cent increased risk of death from a range of causes.[12]

#2 Chicken isn't such a 'healthy' food

In his recent bestseller, *How Not to Die*, the US physician Michael Greger asks the question: 'Which of the following contains more sodium? A serving of beef; an unseasoned serving of roast chicken; a large carton of McDonald's fries, or a serving of salted pretzels.'

The answer is chicken![13]

I couldn't believe it. Admittedly, Greger is writing about US food-industry practices, but ours aren't so different. In the UK as well as elsewhere, the poultry industry commonly injects chicken carcasses with saltwater to inflate their weight artificially, and surprisingly they can still be labelled 100 per cent natural. Consumer Reports have found that some supermarket chickens were so full of sodium that one serving contained a whole day's allowance of salt, and one report showed that some of the chicken on sale in the UK was found to be up to one-fifth water.[14] Isn't that incredible? Far from being a wholesome, nutrition-packed superfood, I discovered that chicken today contains one-third more calories, twice as much fat and a third less protein than it did in 1940. According to researchers at London Metropolitan University, eating 100g of chicken gives you more calories from fat than from protein.[15] And don't get me started on the suffering of the average supermarket chicken. The percentage of 'higher welfare' chickens consumed in the UK is at its lowest ever, according to Jamie Oliver's Food Revolution.[16]

So why is it that there's such a strong cultural belief that chicken and 'white meat' in general are healthy? Speaking personally, my prior conviction stemmed from the idea that white meat contains less fat and fewer calories, but I now know this is rarely the case.

Chicken consumption has been linked to a jump in the risk of pancreatic cancer. For every 50g of chicken eaten, the risk of pancreatic cancer jumps by 72 per cent. Even handling chicken has been linked to an elevated risk,[17] believed to be a result of exposure to poultry cancer-causing viruses. Those who slaughter chickens have nine times the odds of both pancreatic and liver cancer. Even line workers with no contact with live birds have an elevated risk. Something to give you pause for thought next time you catch a tempting aroma of roast chicken.

#3 Eggs can be inflammatory

As I mentioned earlier, eggs are one of the foods that people struggle most to cut out when they switch to a plant-based diet. I know I did. As a bodybuilder, egg-white omelettes were a key part of my weekly diet. Sometimes I'd use six whites in one omelette. But even those consuming fewer eggs find them hard to cut out completely. Eggs are versatile, filling and quick to cook, and in just about every cake out there. But the more knowledge I acquired about eggs, the easier it became to let go of them. Here follows a summary of what I discovered.

Just like female humans, hens have a menstrual cycle that can be daily rather than monthly depending on the time of year. A hen has one ovary that develops fully – the left – and this sends a yolk on its journey. The yolk then forms an egg white as it moves through the reproductive tract into the shell gland. The shell takes around 21 hours to form, and then out pops the egg. Just like the human female menstrual period, this is an unfertilized reproductive cycle, and because of this the egg won't develop into a chick. Thinking about eggs in this way, as a hen's period, helped me adjust to the idea of giving them up!

Aside from this, there's also sound evidence to question the idea of 'eggs' as healthy food to be consumed in abundance. Eggs are loaded with cholesterol as well as saturated fat (70 per cent of calories in one egg is from pure fat). Eggs are also high in a substance called arachidonic acid, an inflammatory compound. The further I get into my nutritional study with eCornell, the more the word 'inflammatory' comes up. In the specific case of eggs, our body can make arachidonic acid itself when our inflammatory response kicks in, but research has questioned the impact of all the excess arachidonic acid that omnivores have in their systems. High egg consumption has also been linked to an elevated risk of several cancers, including breast, bladder, colon, prostate and oral cavity cancers.[18]

#4 It's a fishy business

Until I went vegan, I ate a lot of salmon. Often for breakfast, but it was a go-to staple dinner as well. Whenever I ate it, I felt I was doing myself good. I'd read all about the heart and brain benefits, after all. No food has been more widely trumpeted as 'healthy' than fish. With the claims for heart health and depression (omega-3s in oily fish) now widely known and further hyped by the giant fish-oil supplement industry, most of us accept it as a truth that fish is good for us. Plus, it's delicious. But when I started to dig a little deeper, I discovered the research on omega-3s is contradictory and inconclusive. For example, in a considerable data review in 2018, looking at studies based on data from 100,000 people, there was no conclusive proof that omega-3 supplementation reduced the risk of death.[19]

Aside from this, it's well known that many of the popular types of fish contain high levels of mercury, and that farmed fish such as salmon contains high levels of pesticides as a result of the cramped conditions in which they're raised and the prevalence of lice and other parasites. Antifungals are widely used too, as skin infections spread fast in the jam-packed tanks. And although wild salmon is healthier, one US study found numerous fishmongers passing off (dyed) farmed salmon as wild,[20] so it can be tricky to know what you're buying. Salmon is high in fat (it's made up of around 50 per cent fat), with one fillet containing more cholesterol ounce for ounce than a hamburger. Although much of this is healthy omega-3 fat, overdoing the salmon means you'll be eating a high-fat diet. Finally, all seafood now contains traces of microplastic. Those who consume seafood have been estimated to consume 2,000–11,000 individual pieces of microplastic per year along with their fish and shellfish.[21] Although for the most part this is thought to be relatively harmless, it still made me pause for thought and helped me walk past the smoked salmon at the supermarket without the urge to put it in my trolley.

#5 All that school milk didn't do much for my bones

I held the belief that milk made my bones strong. It was something I understood from my earliest childhood. Milk would give me strong bones because it was full of calcium. As previously mentioned, milk was something I never really enjoyed. It was pretty much like broccoli to me as a child:

I hated it but would drink it because it was good for me, but was it? I dropped milk out of the equation several years before my transition to veganism. I read a few articles claiming that milk was 'not' so good for you and ran with that as I didn't like the stuff anyway. I was still in disbelief though, and secretly thought it had to be. After all, the whole world knows it's the truth, as we're told that milk is good for bone health by our parents, the government, advertising, etc.

So, when I started to look for data to prove that those who consume the most dairy have the strongest bones, I was convinced I'd find concrete evidence. Instead, I found lots of inconclusive studies that didn't prove a significant benefit, and a Swedish study found that increased milk consumption *heightened* the risk of bone fracture.[22] The study's researchers believed this was a consequence of the high levels of D-galactose, a type of sugar in the milk that's known to have an inflammatory effect, increasing oxidative stress. Dairy was never meant for humans but for baby cows. I've always found it fascinating that we human beings are the only species who drink milk from other animals. We're also the only species who continue to drink milk after infancy. Food for thought.

A word on vegan junk

But if you're worried all this is sounding a bit one-sided: omnivores – nil, vegans – 100, I'd like to point out that there are *plenty* of *seriously* unhealthy vegan options too.

Veganism doesn't specify what to eat and so obviously doesn't equate to being healthy. In becoming a vegan, you can make the conscious choice to replace animal food with whole plants, or on the flip side, with nutrient-depleted, processed plant fragments. It's even become trendy to talk about 'dirty vegan junk food', and I've noticed some pop-up markets where stalls selling deep-fried vegan fare have queues snaking around the block. Partly it makes me happy to see vegan fast food in place of fried chicken and burgers, and obviously, the odd junk treat is OK, but I've noticed that it can be tempting to fall into some bad habits when you're making the transition to veganism. You might reach for fries when you wouldn't have before, or eat too many highly processed foods such as Oreos, or nutritionally deficient meat and fake cheese substitutes that are packed with sodium and fat. Or you might overdo it on the refined carbs: white pasta and white bread spring to mind. Again, both are OK in moderation, it's all a question of balance. It's best to scrutinize labels to check how healthy processed vegan food is, as it can vary wildly.

The point I want to make is that you might feel tempted to think that because you're 'being good' by going vegan, you can afford to indulge in lots of unhealthy vegan foods, knowing that you're 'offsetting' any negative health impact with all the extra fruit and veg you're eating. It's easy to assume that as a vegan, you don't have to give 'healthy eating' too much thought. Don't fool yourself that this is the case. There are a whole host of other foods that aren't 'junk' but aren't as nutritious as whole foods either. Meat substitutes (mince but also deli meats) and processed vegan foods such as seitan, made from wheat gluten, fall into this camp. Some of these foods are high in sugar, salt and preservatives, and should be eaten in moderation.

Don't beat yourself up about it though. All of these foods are useful as a way to make your transition to a vegan lifestyle less of a shock or consumed as part of a diet that's otherwise packed with plant-based whole foods, but they shouldn't be regarded as everyday staples.

The typical Western diet that most of us are accustomed to eating is high in saturated and hydrogenated fats, high in animal fats, highly processed, low in complex carbohydrates and also low in fibre, fruits and vegetables. This diet is heavy on everything that prevents optimum health: meat, dairy, white flour, refined sugar and oil. In contrast, the vegan diet plan I recommend focuses not only on the exclusion of animal foods but also the inclusion of whole plants. This is the diet that's kept my father feeling great following his late diagnosis of prostate cancer and his refusal to be treated with chemotherapy. All of my meal recommendations for the diet plan in Chapter 7 are based around foods that haven't been altered from their original state or processed; they've had nothing added or taken away, they're natural and therefore can do the body no harm.

Don't fall into the sugar trap

I can think of a few examples of friends who went vegan and let themselves off the hook on the sugar front. I get it. It can be tough to stick to a vegan diet, so the few 'treats' that are still allowed can be hard to let go of. But (and I'm telling you something you already know, here, but bear with me) if you have a high-sugar diet, you'll be effectively cancelling out much of the benefit of cutting out animal products. It's a credit-debit approach that leaves you at zero.

Sticking to a plant-based whole food diet is best for your health. Whenever you're tempted to reach for the biscuits or give in to an urge for sugary drinks and treats, turn to the list of healthy vegan treats in Chapter 7.

Getting the balance right

As we discovered in the section above on 'vegan junk', going vegan doesn't make you healthier by default (because of the unhealthy animal-based products you're leaving out), although it's easy to assume it should. In fact, eating a balanced vegan diet is harder work and requires more thought and planning than a healthy omnivorous diet.

As a guide for eating well, vegetables and fruit (in a 3:2 ratio) should always make up 50 per cent of your plate. I recommend consuming 0.5kg (1lb) or more of vegetables and fruit daily. Remember to eat a rainbow! Approximately

25 per cent of your plate should be whole grains. Aim for a mix of complex carbohydrates and fibre to ensure you get the required vitamins and minerals you require, and try to limit your intake of refined cereals. The remaining 25 per cent of your plate should be plant protein; good-quality sources include legumes, beans, tofu, tempeh, nuts and seeds. The combination of various sources of plant protein will ensure you get all the essential amino acids you need.

It's easy to eat too little protein, too many processed foods and too narrow a range of food. I found this out to my cost when I went vegan overnight. It was *hard*! I lived on oats, fruit, soya sausages and pasta with tomato sauce for the first few weeks. It left me feeling a little sluggish. It is crucial not to underestimate the amount of thought and consideration you need to put into eating well as a vegan, which is what inspired me to write this book. I want to share all of the mistakes I made, so you don't!

It's essential to compensate for lost nutrients by thinking carefully about vegan replacements (quinoa, peas and lentils instead of chicken, for example). And if you suspect you might be falling short, it might be a good idea to supplement with a multivitamin. I didn't think consciously enough about the balance of macronutrients I was getting in the food I ate, and I paid the price with my energy and wellbeing. I didn't feel my usual self. I didn't feel fit and healthy. Instead, I felt lethargic and at times, low in energy.

Meat alternatives

Here's a question I often get asked about veganism that I find one part hilarious and two parts baffling: 'If you're so against eating animals and their exploitation why do you vegans constantly seek out meat alternatives?'

Maybe it's just me, but I think that's one of the silliest questions out there. I've been eating meat my entire life because, like most of us, it was fed to me as a child, and I acquired a taste for it. I absolutely love the way meat tastes. Little is more delicious than melted cheese toasties, scrambled eggs and salmon on sourdough bread for breakfast, or the fattest chicken breast with crispy skin and gravy for Sunday roast. That was my life.

I'm telling you this to demonstrate that I didn't adopt a plant-based diet on the grounds of taste. I did it for ethical reasons and for moral reasons. I did it to be compassionate, and because I believe it's the right thing to do. I didn't suddenly stop liking the taste of meat. So why wouldn't I seek out vegan alternatives to replace what I was missing?

But in seeking out alternatives, I discovered something. It wasn't meat, I loved particularly. It was the way it was cooked and seasoned that made it delicious. Have you ever cooked or eaten meat without seasoning? Not even salt and/or pepper. It's pretty bland, right? On average I'd say about one in 10 people I've had this conversation with say they'd enjoy the taste of such bland meat. The others, like myself, were quick to identify that without additional flavourings (seasoning, gravy or sauce), they really wouldn't enjoy meat at all. It's the texture and seasonings most of us genuinely enjoy. So, if I can get that same texture and consistency in plant-based products (that are better for me and don't harm my body), and then apply that same seasoning that I'd use if I were cooking meat, why on earth wouldn't I do that? Wouldn't you?

Fake meats tend either to be made from a highly processed soy, pea or wheat gluten base, or fermented edible mould. None of these is brilliant from a health point of view, although they won't do you any harm in moderation. If I had to pick one out as the healthiest, I'd say pea-protein based meats are best as they contain all nine essential amino acids (although it's low in methionine). I struggled to find any bad review on it. Tofu again has mixed reviews. It is an unfermented soy product that some people choose to avoid as its heavy consumption could disrupt your hormone levels and tofu products often come from GM crops. That being said, I personally will have tofu every now and then, but like everything else, I think it's essential to be mindful about it. Have the information and make an informed choice.

The lowdown on B12

In the 12-week plan, I recommend supplementing with vitamin B12 because after 'Where do you get your protein from?', the second most frequently asked question I hear is:

'If a vegan diet is natural, why will a person following a vegan lifestyle die if they fail to supplement vitamin B12?'

The fact is, people can and do die from nutritional deficiencies of all kinds regardless of their food consumption. But there are many nutrients that vegans might need to pay more attention to than meat-eaters, just as there are many other nutrients many meat-eaters are more likely to be lacking in than vegans. B12 is clearly a big concern for vegans, who are far more likely to be deficient in it. It was the first thing brought to my attention on becoming a vegan. I met an old friend of my mother's, who was a vegetarian. Her friend who happened to be a vegan turned up, and we got chatting. One of the first things she said to me was 'Make sure you take a B12 supplement. There are no sources of B12 that are vegan.' It's something anyone considering switching to a vegan diet needs to read up on because people CAN (and do) die from a B12 deficiency.

The question that always baffled me was this: how can B12 be a problem for vegans when it originates from vegan sources (i.e. the soil)? I discovered in the course of my research that B12 is a vitamin like no other. I learned we only require incredibly small amounts – as little as 10mg a day – and it can take as long as five years to show symptoms of deficiency. It's the *only* vitamin that doesn't seem to be available from a varied, whole food, plant-based diet together with sun exposure. That being said, several foods are fortified with vitamin B12, including some varieties of plant milk, breakfast cereals and the one most love or hate, Marmite. I love Marmite! The reason B12 is said to be a problem for vegans – at least in the UK and other so-called 'advanced' nations – isn't because it's not present in our fruit and veg, but because the majority of produce is grown in ways that end up totally removing the vitamin. B12 is in the soil and, interestingly, all B12 does, in fact, *originate* from vegan sources. When animals eat grass, for example, they absorb it, and we, in turn, benefit when we eat them! But the chemicals used to grow fruit and vegetables farmed for human consumption need to be aggressively washed off, and with them, all traces of soil are lost.

Are you immediately at risk? Well, no. In fact, I learned on my plant-based nutrition course that it can take many years – because of the tiny daily amount of B12 we need, and our residual stores – for symptoms of a deficiency to show. It's common for former meat and dairy consumers to have stored up enough B12 in their systems to keep them going for five, 10 years or even longer. This fact explains how so many vegans can rightly claim to be completely healthy despite not consuming any form of animal products, fortified vegan products or supplements. It doesn't mean it's safe to do so, though, particularly for those who may not have built up this safety net.

So, what's the best B12 supplement to go for? Head to the health food store, and you'll be confronted by shelves of them. My initial reaction was to reach for the cheapest one – they all did the same thing, I figured, so why spend extra money on them? However, since then, I've learned more about nutrition, completing my plant-based course, and I discovered that our bodies can only absorb a tiny amount of the vitamin. So, selecting supplements with high doses of B12 is pointless. In fact, according to Dr Colin T Campbell, you need only the tiniest amount of B12 daily – about 2.4mcg. He says a multivitamin should provide more than enough.

A word of caution about supplements

Overdosing on nutrients is pretty much impossible when you're eating real foods. You simply can't consume them in the quantities that would make you seriously ill. Try eating 9kg (20lb) of spinach, drinking 6 litres of water or a bottle of vodka in one go! All of these could be fatal, even the spinach (it's the oxalic acid that would get you). However, if you're consuming nutrients in pill form, or if your recommended daily dose of folic acid is contained in a single serving of cereal, is it safe to eat a whole box, while also taking folic acid supplements, and eating fortified bread? Over months or years, eating too many fortified foods and taking supplements could mean you get too much of a good thing. Not to be recommended. That's why I advocate whole foods wherever possible, cooking from scratch and avoiding supplements except for B12 or a multivitamin containing B12.

Chapter 4

Do Good, Feel Good

Let's focus on the positive motivation for going vegan. When you stop consuming animal products, you're doing a great thing for the environment. You're also choosing to stand up and say that you no longer want to benefit from the death or suffering of any animals. That should make you feel great! It's important to celebrate this conviction and hold on to it, which can be hard if you're surrounded by people mocking you or questioning your choice to do something different.

On my first day as a vegan, I felt on top of the world! When I woke up at first light, I was overcome with a sense of joy. Simply knowing that I was no longer contributing to the pain and suffering of animals lifted my spirit. It was kind of like an awakening. The recognition of my own dysfunction up to that point was liberating and gave me a sense of inner peace I'd never experienced before. The eggs and salmon I'd always started my day with were now a thing of the past, but my breakfast oats, banana, nuts and seeds, with unsweetened almond milk gave me everything I needed to kickstart my day.

I was working at Battersea fire station at the time, and when I told my fellow firefighters about my new lifestyle, they were quick to use it as an opportunity to make fun of me. I'd expected that: bacon sandwiches wafted under my nose, biting into chicken drumsticks in front of me and saying: 'Don't you want some of this, Ed?' There's a lot of banter in the fire service, and I was fully aware that adopting a plant-based diet would be regarded as readymade material. Mostly, it was pretty funny. But not all of it felt light-hearted. There was the odd angry comment too, and I was regularly invited to enter into debate with colleagues to defend my choice. I was told repeatedly that humans had evolved to be carnivores, and that we need to eat meat, even though I'd explained my decision in personal terms. I wasn't expecting to convert anyone else or to tell other people how to eat, and I didn't want to get drawn into endless, circular arguments with my bacon-loving colleagues.

A few of my buddies were more supportive and quietly told me they admired my willpower and wished they had the same. Or they'd confide that they too had moral concerns themselves about the way animals were treated by the farming industry. These occasional, positive responses helped strengthen my resolve. Alongside the belief in what I was doing, it meant I was able to zone out all the negative comments and stay true to my decision. I felt good inside about my choice.

Ten do-good, feel-good reasons to go vegan

I kept a list in my head of all the reasons why I was going vegan, and I'd check in with them whenever I'd struggle. I'd like to share an expanded list with you and suggest you cut it out and put it somewhere you'll see it every day to remind you of the do-good, feel-good motivators. Here they are:

1. You'll save the lives of (on average) 10 animals a month.

2. Vegans have a 43 per cent lower risk of obesity than carnivores.[1]

3. It's the single most significant lifestyle change you can make to reduce your carbon footprint, reducing your dietary footprint by up to 73 per cent if you were previously a meat-eater.[2] Going vegan trumps buying an electric car and cutting down on flights. Going vegan doesn't just reduce greenhouse gases, it massively reduces land use, water use, hormone and antibiotic contamination of the food chain and the negative agricultural side effects of soil acidification.

4. Going vegan cuts your overall cancer risk by 19 per cent[3–4]. Excluding meat from your diet also slashes the risk of some other forms of cancer by far more (up to 45 per cent), including bladder and bowel cancer.[5]

5. Vegans weigh less. In a study of 12 different types of diet, those who ate a vegan diet saw the most dramatic weight loss.

6. Your skin will glow. Dairy consumption has been linked with acne risk, and increasing your antioxidants, with all the fruit and veg you'll be eating, will help fight oxidative damage that leads to skin ageing.[6]

7. Because so many unhealthy and processed foods contain animal products, you'll significantly reduce the number of unhealthy foods you might otherwise be tempted to snack on.

8. In a recent online poll, 64 per cent of participants stated they have increased energy and vitality as a vegan compared to their omnivorous days.[7] I've certainly noticed increased energy in the bedroom and relationships.

9. The CO_2 figures are simple. If you eat a meat-rich diet, you'll be producing 7.2kg of carbon dioxide emissions. Vegetarian and pescatarian diets result in 3.8kg per day, whereas vegan diets result in 2.9kg per day.[8] Combined climate-change emissions for meat-eating alone were calculated at 18 per cent of the total by the United Nations. Many argue this is a gross underestimate, with one report by World Bank scientists in 2009 revised the figure up to 51 per cent.[9]

10. Veganism is compassion in action. It's compassionate in the broadest sense of the word, encompassing compassion towards all other species and life forms with which we share this planet.

Awakening to compassion

When I decided to become a vegan, moral and emotional conviction kicked in pretty much overnight. I had an epiphany when I watched the documentary *Earthlings* for the first time, and I knew there was no going back for me. It wasn't just the cruelty and compassion that became important to me, it was the whole picture: environmental, moral and social. I couldn't cut my meat consumption gradually because I couldn't bear the thought of eating it at all. I literally went from eating meat at any time of the day, not caring about recycling, or my carbon footprint or the impact of my food choices on my daughter's generation, to feeling painfully aware of all of it, all the time. I felt so guilty about all the damage I'd inflicted on the world, and all the animals that had died to feed me.

The more I started to look into the meat industry and think about farming and slaughter, and the impact of the food I'd been eating (on the environment, my body, and most of all, on the animals) it was as if I was jolted awake.

I care about animals and the environment, and I believe in equality for all living beings. The scale of the slaughter I'd willingly benefited from suddenly became profoundly upsetting for me. Online, I found statistics that totalled the average meat-eater's animal consumption over a lifetime: I discovered the average US omnivore, for example, consumes 11 cows, 27 pigs, 2,400 chickens, 80 turkeys, 30 sheep and

4,500 fish throughout a lifetime.[10] Guiltily, I wondered what my 'average' had been – what with all the extra protein I'd eaten to support my bodybuilding regime. I began to visualize all the animals I'd mindlessly consumed. Then I wondered about the butterfly-effect consequences: the greenhouse gas emissions, the hormones in the water supply and the colossal waste of resources. Mainly, though I thought about the suffering: the cramped cages, the lack of sunlight, the trauma of animals seeing their fellow creatures slaughtered and sensing the same was about to happen to them.

On social media one day, I stumbled across a video a friend had shared of the Buddhist monk, sometimes called the 'happiest man in the world', Matthieu Ricard talking about his reasons for being vegan. In the video interview,[11] he explained that veganism is a compassionate response to the 'instrumentalized' slaughter of animals, which he compared to genocide. He also pointed out that making a choice to switch to veganism is 'so simple, it can be done instantly'. He says, 'It's not an extreme perspective. It's a reasonable, compassionate point of view.'

Particularly with the publication of the Oxford University study mentioned earlier, a vegan diet is beginning to look like the only sustainable way to eat for the future of our planet. This means that many people who aren't convinced by the compassionate argument alone are now considering veganism based on the environmental debate. This is great news. Motivation and 'whys' come in a wide range of flavours. The important thing is to identify the motivation that makes the most sense to you.

The environmental 'why'

To sum up the key stats from the Oxford study, looking at 40,000 farms worldwide, lead researcher Joseph Poore, who turned vegan himself a year into the study, said:

> *A vegan diet is probably the single biggest way to reduce your impact on planet earth… It is far bigger than cutting down on your flights or buying an electric car. Avoiding consumption of animal products delivers far better environmental benefits than trying to purchase sustainable meat and dairy.*[12]

I began to imagine a world where everyone was vegan, and there was no longer a need to farm animals. So much destruction could be avoided, including the mowing down of rainforests, which continues to lead to the mass extinction of wildlife. Without meat and dairy consumption, experts estimate that global farmland use could be massively reduced by more than 75 per cent and still feed the world. Even for those who protest that they eat high-welfare meat, the sums just don't seem to add up. Inevitably, I found myself thinking, huge-scale environmental destruction and a sky-high carbon footprint is too much of a price to pay for the purpose of taste, habit, tradition and culture. Meat and dairy provide

18 per cent of calories and 37 per cent of protein but use a whopping 83 per cent of farmland while producing 60 per cent of agriculture's greenhouse gas emissions.[13] Basically, it's really inefficient in terms of energy and resources in and calories and protein out.

Cows are a great example. They are what's known as 'ruminants' due to having to chew and then ferment food before digesting it. This is a lengthy process and makes them inefficient in converting food to energy. Almost none of what they eat goes into their bloodstream. This means the number of resources it takes to create a single meal of beef is off the scale. Beef production relies on high water consumption and lots of water pollution, as well as a whole load of grass, grains and other food. It's wasteful because those same resources could have fed several families plant-based meals, cutting out the 'middle-man' as it were. In terms of land use, beef production relies on land to grow plant-based food for the cattle, and grazing land. In many parts of the world, cattle farming is the leading cause of deforestation. Acres of rainforest are being cut down every year, with a substantial resulting loss to the affected ecosystems. Birds, insects and rare plants are being lost so that we can eat more burgers. Over time, this land becomes overgrazed and nutritionally depleted. It can take years to recover.

What about that rumour that most of this deforestation is due to planting vegetable crops? This is something I've heard a few times, particularly as a response to my suggestions that a vegan diet is less harmful to the environment. I was concerned that perhaps the environmental benefits of veganism were too good to be true. But when I looked into it in more depth, I discovered that although there was some truth in deforestation making way for plant-based crops, the story didn't end there because the majority is either for livestock or to grow fodder.[14] Already one-third of the available land on the planet (not including areas covered with ice) is used for these purposes. In the USA, 13 million hectares were being used for plants, whereas 302 million were being used for livestock. This situation is worsening with increasing meat and dairy consumption worldwide. One of the most staggering statistics I came across told me that 86 per cent of the world's land animals were now livestock farmed for human consumption.[15]

In addition to all this, the vast amount of animal waste and eye-watering volume of cattle farts produce methane (one of the most harmful greenhouse gases) in gut-churning quantities that are contributing to global warming.[16] Animal waste leads to pollution problems and contaminates neighbouring farms and often the water supply.

I know I've said this already, but I'll repeat it. If you're an omnivore, you could do more to save the planet just by giving up meat and dairy than if you sold your car and stopped taking plane flights. This isn't something most people realize.

Still sceptical? Let me ask you something. How much water do you think it takes to grow plants? I'll tell you. It can vary from 32 litres (8½ gallons) to produce 0.5kg (1lb) of potatoes, to 104 litres (27½ gallons) to produce 0.5kg (1lb) of rice. How much water do you think a cow needs, for us to get 0.5kg (1lb) of beef to eat? Do you think it's at the high end of that scale? If you do, you're very wrong. It's nearly 11,000 litres (2,900 gallons). That's 100 times the amount of water for the same quantity of food.[17]

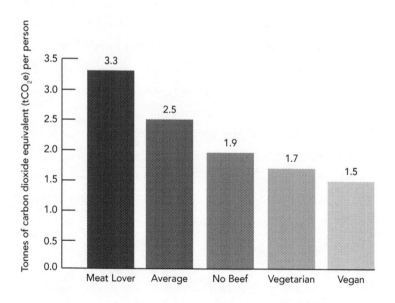

Comparative carbon 'foodprints' (tCO$_2$e per person) based on average food production emissions for the USA.[18]

As a parent, the harsh reality of these statistics hit home. I understood it was my responsibility to do whatever I could to safeguard the planet for my daughter's generation.

When I recognized the environmental upside of transitioning to veganism, it was a real lightbulb moment. Whereas before, my attitude like most people was: 'Whatever I do won't really make a difference,' I realize now that this apathy was based on a false justification. I'd chosen ignorance and laziness over knowledge and change; I'd chosen selfish over selfless.

Once I started to consider the devastating consequences of my actions, I became passionate that by becoming a vegan, I really could 'be the change'. It's not just the harming of animals we need to consider, but ourselves, our Earth and future generations. Civilization depends on animals, plants and micro-organisms that supply vital ecosystems. Bee and insect populations are an obvious example. Another is woodland and forest. We mass-produce billions of land animals and with that comes trillions of tons of manure. Where does it all go? As you can imagine, there's no way it can all be contained. Some get in the waterways, there's run off to the crops, or they're sometimes putting untreated or partially treated faeces-contaminated water directly on to the crops, which has huge public health implications.

The compassionate 'why'

I'm going to hit you with a few facts about animal products that I think would give even the most committed carnivore pause for thought. Before I do that though, I want you to think about 'humane' slaughter for a moment. Slaughterhouses are the scene of substantial psychological cruelty to animals, as well as physical abuse and torture. No humane act takes place there.

All animals tend to be slaughtered when and where they reach the best price, so animals at one end of the UK are often transported hundreds of miles for slaughter. The more I discovered about the industrial-scale slaughter of animals, watching documentaries and reading books on the subject, the bigger my compassion towards animals grew. Worldwide, it's common for farm animals to be packed into rail containers or lorries and transported hundreds of miles, sometimes across continents, for slaughter. The conditions of transportation are brutally inhumane. Animals are packed in, standing in their own urine and waste for days, with no access to water. When they reach their final destination, they're scared to dismount. These animals are very intuitive. They can feel it; they know what's coming.

And even when animals are used, rather than killed by us, I find the cruelty mind-boggling. Cows need to be pregnant to produce milk. The dairy industry repeatedly impregnates cows, starting when they're as young as one year, to encourage milk production. Their newborn calves on each occasion are taken away at birth, to prevent them from drinking the milk that's intended for human consumption. This is traumatic for the mother as well as the calf. Most female calves will be raised to be milk-making machines as their mothers were, and male calves are often slaughtered within 48 hours and sold as veal, as some breeds of dairy cattle aren't suitable for beef. Calves that do survive will often call for their mother (and similarly, the mother will call for her lost calf) for days. I saw this in one of the films I watched, and the sadness of both mother and calf was so real I could feel it. Dairy cows are encouraged to produce milk at around 10 times the natural rate, which means their udders are overly heavy, uncomfortable and prone to infection, causing pus and blood in the milk they produce.

I don't know about you, but I'd rather spare the poor cows altogether. They really have drawn the short straw. A healthy cow's life expectancy is 20–25 years; however, due to the physical and emotional suffering they endure, they aren't suitable for milk production for more than five years, after which most are slaughtered for beef.

Most pigs in the UK are intensively reared on farms and are kept in small crates. Female pigs, who would nest in the wild, finding somewhere quiet to give birth, are forced to give birth on concrete floors. The crates restrict movement so much; they can't reach their piglets properly to nuzzle them. The concrete floors and crate bars cause pressure sores. To keep pigs in such confined spaces, large quantities of antibiotics and other medication are required.

In the UK, 94 per cent of the 900 million chickens slaughtered each year are reared on factory farms, while in the USA, the figure is 99.9 per cent.[19] Chicken and egg farming are seriously big business, and broiler and laying chickens experience some of the worst conditions of all farmed animals. But hang on a minute, you might think that 'battery farming' was banned in the UK years ago? You're right in one sense: single-cell cages were banned in 2012, but instead, farmers were allowed to replace them with 'colony cages' with one perch, filling their 5m long by 2m wide spaces with up to 80 birds.

Broiler chickens are bred to produce as much meat as possible, so in their cramped conditions, their bodies often grow too big for their bones, which may break under the strain. Laying hens are fed a special diet to encourage them to lay up to 300 eggs per year per bird, a load that takes its toll on their wings and bones, as the calcium to make shells depletes their own. Male chicks of laying hens are killed at birth. Hens who are too sick or old to lay at the required rate are slaughtered by being shackled upside down and having their heads dipped in electrified water.

Sheep tend to be reared outside, in fields, so they get to graze naturally, but this also means they often have no shelter from the Sun or flooding. They are often impregnated by the insertion of an electric probe with semen while the animal is held in a rack. This is uncomfortable and distressing. Hormones are used to encourage sheep to produce more lambs than they would naturally, and to give birth even in midwinter, which means more of their lambs die, and when more than the two they can suckle are born, the others are taken away to be bottle-fed.

I share all of this with you not to scaremonger, but in the hope that it might inspire you to question your habits (if you currently consume meat and/or dairy) and to stand by your choice if you've already made the switch.

To me, identifying as an ethical vegan represents strength. Having the courage of my convictions to stand up for what I believe to be right; to change my habits, and to go against the grain socially. Being vegan to me means being authentic and living in a way that's in tune with my core values.

Veganism is kindness. It's one of the greatest gifts that can both change a life and save a life. To get spiritual about it, kindness is a manifestation of love. To love others as you love yourself. To recognize that just as we do, animals feel fear, love, happiness, pain, suffering and misery. Just like us, they have every desire to live and to be free.

I remember feeling really moved when I saw an interview with the US mixed martial artist Mac Danzig in the *Forks Over Knives* documentary. He talked about his experience as a teenager, seeing a pig on its way to slaughter:

> *I remember seeing a truck on the interstate filled with pigs all headed to the slaughterhouse. One of them made eye contact with me for a while. It was one of the saddest moments I can remember. There was so much intelligence and spirit in him, and here he was, being sent to a terrible death.*[20]

As I continue on my path and learn more, my personal definition of veganism expands. What was once a decision purely based on animal welfare has now become so much more. I've totally changed my mindset as a result of discovering new levels of compassion and rethinking my attitude towards animals. I don't resent any of the 'sacrifices' involved in being a vegan. Instead, I feel a tremendous amount of guilt that I spent the first 30 years of my life utterly oblivious to the amount of suffering I caused animals – something I didn't give a second thought. It's as if I considered wearing leather and eating chicken as my birthright as a human being. But as soon as I began to really think about where my food and clothes had come from, I found it profoundly upsetting that I'd felt no association with animals, even when I'd been wearing their skin.

This is true for most of us. The industrialized, 'hidden away' farming industry and manufacturing of food and clothes make it easier than ever to consider the unsavoury realities behind the treatment of animals by human beings. It takes bravery to face up to it, but I believe the rewards are more than worth it.

Why vegan feels so good

In her book *The Power of Meaning*, the US journalist Emily Esfahani Smith argues that fulfilment in life comes about through living a life of meaning and purpose. She says when we feel our daily life is out of step with our deep values, depression, anxiety and feelings of powerlessness can take hold. Her suggestion that 'the ability to find purpose in the day-to-day tasks of living and working goes a long way towards building meaning', really resonates with me. For me, veganism is an excellent example of this. We all need to eat and turning it into a conscious choice is a way to create a sense of purpose and positivity about the way we're living, day to day.

The 2014 documentary *Cowspiracy*, which I binge-watched back to back after *Earthlings*, is about the environmental impact of the beef industry. In an interview after it came out, its director Kip Anderson said that compassionate veganism is transforming public perception of the lifestyle transition:

Whereas before, veganism may have been viewed like you were giving up something, now it's been reframed as what you gain: you gain health, you gain a greater sense of living in bounds with your values, you gain all the environmental benefits.[21]

It's helpful to commit to taking this positive, empowering view of a vegan lifestyle if you want to stick with it. Whenever you feel tempted to revert to old ways of eating or water down your reasons for changing your diet in conversation, remind yourself of what you're gaining and why it is you feel a vegan lifestyle is the best choice for you.

Based on current trends, with developing countries experiencing the biggest jumps in population and switching to more Western diets where meat forms the basis of almost every meal, things are likely to get worse before they get better. All this consumption inevitably means that more forests are destroyed, more pollution is generated and more problems are being stored up for our children's futures. This puts the onus on us in the West to do what we can. And by going vegan we're taking a positive step towards a more sustainable, compassionate future.

Chapter 5

Where to Start?

So, you're still with me. I'm going to go ahead and assume that this means you've decided to take the plunge. To make the switch to the vegan lifestyle.

If you want this to be a dietary change you can stick with, a word of warning. I've lost track of the number of people who have told me that despite setting out with the best of intentions, they struggled to sustain it. If you try to make the switch overnight as I did, you're more likely to fall at the first hurdle. This is purely because it'll probably feel surprisingly tough to transform both the nutrient balance (by cutting out animal proteins) and the type of diet (by switching to whole foods only), at the same time. Anything that feels like deprivation is going to be hard to stick to, so the objective is to make the transition sustainable, and think of it as a positive lifestyle shift rather than a restrictive regime.

Don't think of it as a diet

This is a big one. Although many of those starting out on a diet are doing so for the right reasons: to improve their health, and take their wellbeing into their own hands, the very word 'diet' may be linked to thoughts of deprivation, which is certainly not the message I'm trying to convey! I have great news: eating The Fit Vegan diet doesn't require you to reduce your food intake massively, nor does it require you to get rid of foods you deem tasty.

On my plant-based nutrition course, I learned that our brains are conditioned to react if our calorie or fat intake drops significantly. When we feel hungry, our body responds by releasing more of the 'hunger hormone', leptin, to stimulate our appetites to restore the balance. This explains why much of the time, depriving ourselves only makes our bodies crave the lost calories. Where weight loss is a key objective, I recommend clients try not to think about that, reassuring them the extra pounds will fall away as a side effect of whole food plant-based eating. When you're eating a plant-based, whole food diet and exercising, you mustn't place any further restrictions on what you're eating. That translates as no constantly counting calories, or deliberately avoiding the high-calorie, high-fat foods you can eat (avocado for example). Instead, I want to ensure that your new plant-based diet feels exciting, delicious and filling, giving you the energy you need to train your way to a strong, lean and healthy body.

So how should you set about transitioning to veganism? Follow these pointers:

Keep it simple

I wouldn't recommend you throw yourself in at the deep end. Healthy vegan convenience foods (readymade beanburgers, meat substitutes, pre-prepared grains and marinated tofu) are lifesavers for those who are time-pressed or don't have the inclination to spend ages soaking pulses or creating curry bases from scratch. It's so important to be realistic about what is likely to work for you. I'm not saying an overnight switch to plant-based, from-scratch meals can't be done, but unless your diet is already relatively clean and you're an enthusiastic cook, be realistic. Don't overcomplicate things by attempting to follow elaborate recipes with loads of ingredients you've never used before. The recipes I've created in Chapter 7 are designed to replicate everyday omnivorous favourites. There are a few more adventurous ideas, but nothing that takes longer than 20 minutes to prepare. Don't forget, if something feels too much like hard work, you'll be far more likely to give up on it. Make it easy for yourself. Once you've got a few simple, delicious vegan dishes under your belt, you can branch out to try more complicated and unfamiliar things.

Luckily for you, thanks to veganism becoming much more mainstream, a lot more products are labelled as such now. They have the certified vegan logo or are labelled suitable for vegans. Granted, it might seem frustrating or time-consuming to check everything at first, especially when you're used to throwing the usual suspects on your shopping list into your basket, but after a few weeks, it becomes second nature. Embrace the change and understand that you're just being mindful about what you're putting in your body and trying to live a life in which you cause the least amount of harm possible.

Don't think all or nothing

If you've been vegan-curious for a while, you may have come across some of the many documentaries and books on the subject. Watching them can inspire an urge to make a radical and immediate change. On one level, this is great, but it can lead to you piling the pressure on yourself to cut out all animal products overnight. Although I understand the appeal of going cold turkey, I don't recommend it for most people. It's worth considering whether you might have more chance of long-term success if you cut back on animal products slowly. I recommend this particularly if you're cooking for children (more of this in Chapter 8), as I know from experience that children's dietary preferences can be rigid, and any change can cause a whole lot of stress for parents and protests from kids. Introducing new foods slowly and incrementally seems to work better than expecting children to switch from sausage and mash to tofu stir fry without so much as a backward glance.

When I come to think of it, we grown-ups aren't that different. Slowly but surely is a sound principle to follow in most areas of life, whether it's relationships, fitness or study. It's no coincidence that Veganuary stats from a poll conducted on the 60,000 people who took part in Veganuary in January 2017 found that those most likely to remain vegan six months later were those who were already vegetarian at the beginning. If you're not ready to go full vegan, try eating a veggie diet for a few months, then you'll be in a better position to give veganism a good go.

For some clients, I recommend cooking two or three plant-based meals a week. I might recommend more for some and fewer for others, depending on their goals, current lifestyle, situation and readiness to change. I encourage them to take their favourite meals and replicate them using plant-based substitutes where they'd typically use meat. For example, replacing the egg pasta and mince beef of a traditional Bolognese with pea mince and whole wheat pasta, or replacing the chicken in a stir fry with tofu. Within my meal plans, you'll find various options that I'm sure will tickle your taste buds while showing you the power of healthy, plant-based nutrition.

Get organized

Meal planning is key to a smooth transition to plant-based whole food eating. Most of the time, when clients fall off the wagon, it's at 8 p.m. on a Sunday night when the only thing in the freezer is an old, meat-based ready meal. Who can blame them for reaching for it? Temporary phases in life that are busier than usual, and feeling generally overtired and overloaded, are also potential flashpoints where willpower can fade. You're only human, after all. The best way to ensure you don't get caught out is to plan your meals in advance and book shopping deliveries ahead of time. Making sure you have quick, nutritious and appealing plant-based options to hand is essential. The recipes in Chapter 7 are an excellent place to start and investing in the plant-ready-kitchen staples (*see p.186*) will ensure you can turn whatever you have into something extra delicious.

Double the benefit

You might question whether it's a good idea to try radically changing your diet and taking up a new exercise regime at the same time. But that's precisely what I recommend you do in the 12-week plan. But rather than looking at it as double the pressure, I wholeheartedly believe it's actually your secret motivational weapon. Exercising will boost your mood, your self-esteem and your willpower. It will make you much more likely to stick with the dietary changes. Simultaneously, your healthy new plant-based diet will give you the energy and endurance you need to fuel your workouts.

Progressive transition

You have several options if you decide to transition slowly from your current eating habits to a fully vegan diet.

If you're an omnivore, try going veggie (making a conscious effort to up your consumption of plant-based whole foods while you're at it) for a few weeks and see how you feel. Two to three nights a week, cook a vegan meal. Next, cut out dairy, and finally, try ditching the eggs, all the time increasing the number of vegan meals you eat. Don't be self-critical about taking your time and applaud the positive impact your new diet will be having on your carbon footprint and health. I was reading up on zero waste recently and stumbled across this inspiring saying: 'We don't need a few people doing zero waste perfectly, we need everyone doing it a bit.' It's the same with veganism, which is why campaigns like Veganuary are excellent news, even if not everyone manages to stick to their new diet long-term.

If you're a veggie or an omnivore with cast-iron willpower and no extra stresses or pressures in your life that might derail your new regime, go ahead and go plant-based vegan. Be mindful of avoiding the pitfalls I mentioned at the beginning of this chapter and choose meals from the easy vegan meal planner in Chapter 7. Buy yourself a wall planner and write your meals and workouts on it to make things easy for yourself (and to make yourself accountable). Put workouts and meal plans in your phone or computer calendar, too. Batch cook when you can to make sure there are a few emergency vegan meals in the freezer to avoid the 8 p.m. on Sunday lasagne trap.

Setting goals

I'm a big believer in setting goals. They help you target your energy in the right direction. When you have goals that are authentic and meaningful to you, and just challenging enough, they're incredibly motivating. Goals help you become more present and more conscious of the choices you make day to day. They are a great way to make your deepest intentions deliberate. I'd like to help you set some personal lifestyle goals that will help keep you on track.

I'd go as far as to say that setting goals is essential if you want to succeed with your new plant-based eating plan. No goals mean no control. Goals make you accountable to yourself, and failure to set them means you risk failing yourself. Don't leave it down to chance, get planning.

I remember learning about SMART goals way back in school. Since then, I've lived by the rule that to motivate and inspire, a goal had to pass the SMART test. SMART goals are:

S: be **specific** about exactly what it is you want to achieve.

M: make sure your goal is **measurable** by breaking it into smaller elements. So, sticking to a plant-based lifestyle might mean eating seven servings of fruit and veg a day, and cutting out dairy to improve your skin and processed food to increase your energy.

A: the goal should be an **attainable** aspiration. Be wary of goals that are likely to be almost impossible to achieve.

R: I'm all about keeping it **real**. You know yourself and your willpower. Don't jump to plant-based eating 24/7 unless you know you can maintain it. I love the saying: 'You have to crawl before you can walk.' And I'd like to add: 'It's important to enjoy the crawl while you're at it.'

T: for a goal to have the best chance of success, you must make it **time-specific**. Give yourself a schedule, and the same goes for your smaller, measurable goals along the way too. The timeline should be flexible to help you maintain morale and positivity. Don't beat yourself up if you don't hit them all, but just knowing you've set them will galvanize you to stick with the (new) programme.

When you think about your goal, whether it's a small element of a bigger-picture goal or a milestone, make sure you anchor the feeling of what success would feel and look like to you. Identify what you feel, see and hear when your goal has become a reality. Use visualization to imagine yourself looking healthy, fit and happy, running about with your children, playing tennis or running 10K or a marathon. Whatever works for you.

To get you started, set a big-picture goal by writing down your vision and then breaking it down into achievable, measurable chunks. So, for example: 'I want to become a fit vegan' may be your vision. Now it's time to break it down:

I want to become a fit vegan by learning about veganism, identifying with my reasons for making the change, learning new and simple recipes to prepare plant-based meals three times a week and following TFV 12-week vegan fitness regime.

A note on going cold turkey

I understand that the thought or decision to go cold turkey with an overnight transition is so tempting. Especially if you're transitioning for ethical reasons. I watched *Earthlings* and witnessed the atrocities that innocent beings were suffering at our hands. There was no way I could continue consuming animal products, so I felt an overnight transition was my only choice. I didn't even ask myself whether I'd be able to stick with it. Looking back, that was a massive gamble. Yes, fortunately for me, my health and animals worldwide, it paid off. But why gamble if you don't have to. Just like real life, before placing your bet, you'd first look at the odds. That's precisely what you have to do with transitioning to veganism. Look at the odds and be really honest with yourself. Your likelihood to succeed at sticking with an overnight all-or-nothing change is the sum of your willpower:

- Have you stuck with similar radical changes in the past, despite the temptation to revert to your old ways?

- Your motivation – how much do you want to do this?

- Your integrity – to what extent do you tend to live by your morals or values?

- Your why – what is your reason for doing this, and how passionately do you feel about it?

As human beings, we've been programmed since birth, by our parents, society, schooling, and many other influences and factors. We have been conditioned to believe we need meat, and that there's little more nourishing than cow's milk. We treat ourselves with artisan cheese and creamy milk chocolate. Can you really expect decades of programming to be undone overnight? Ensure you don't set yourself up to fail by acknowledging the forces at play here and thinking in advance about how you'll manage them. We've all experienced trying to abstain from something we're absolutely craving. This horrible feeling is so hard to withstand because our brains are crying out for the dopamine hit we've come to associate with the 'fix' – whatever it might be. It's stressful to sit tight until the impulse passes. For most people, I believe that a gradual transition eliminates this kind of pressure, as you can phase out your old diet as you introduce the new one. Having said that, if you're convinced you have what it takes, go ahead and go full vegan today.

Six tips for a smooth transition

1. Learn as much as you can about veganism but do it slowly and methodically. Don't bombard yourself with information, as it'll be hard to retain. Instead, gradually equip yourself with the knowledge that will empower you to progress. As you do your research, make a conscious effort to define your personal 'why'. Read the books and watch the documentaries listed in the Resources (*see p.237*), but ration yourself to a couple a week.

2. You can also connect to the vegan community online by joining Facebook groups, reading blogs and following vegan influencers on Instagram and Twitter. Tapping into a network of like-minded people will help you share the journey.

3. Focus on what you're adding to your diet rather than what you're taking away. With a gradual transition, that's easier to achieve. Enjoy eating a greater variety of fruit and veg, and more whole grains, nuts, seeds and legumes. Focus on the fact that you're now getting more of the nutrients and vitamins your body requires to perform at its optimum level. You'll soon start feeling the benefits of increased plant consumption. This is a significant incentive for upping your vegan days (e.g. from three days a week to four, etc.).

4. Start reading ingredient lists and discover precisely what you're eating. With my overnight transition, there were a

few things I ate in the first couple of months that I didn't know weren't vegan as the animal-derived ingredient wasn't obvious to me or was something I wasn't aware of. Examples that spring to mind are readymade stir-fry sauces that contained Thai fish sauce, crisps that had traces of milk in the flavouring and a takeaway vegetable curry that had been cooked with ghee. I rarely eat bread, but on the occasions that I do, it'll be wholemeal wraps or wholemeal pitta. Some of my vegan friends who consume white bread would unknowingly consume an ingredient commonly known as L-Cysteine or E920, an amino acid used as a flour improver and permitted for use in all biscuits, bread and cakes, excluding wholemeal products.[1] L-Cysteine is produced from pig bristles, feathers and sometimes even human hair.

5. Looking back, the thing that helped me the most, second to my constant identifying with my reasoning for the transition, was always having food to hand. Try not to let yourself get to the place where you're famished with no vegan snacks at hand. Preparation is key to this. Make a list of your favourite snacks and ensure you always have something handy so that you're never caught off-guard when cravings kick in.

6. Think about the timings of your meals around your work-outs. Ensure you eat something 30–60 minutes before you exercise so your body has glucose to burn. In the past, I've worked out first thing in the morning on an empty

stomach. Although I'd sometimes have a great workout at this time, I often found myself running on empty. I believe now that it was adrenalin and determination that got me through as I'd feel light-headed and low in energy shortly after concluding the workout. Instead of my body burning glucose, it was breaking down muscle, which I later came to discover as my progression came to a halt. Now you get to learn from my mistakes, fuelling up before and after training to maximize energy and afterburn. Check out the list of pre- and post-workout snacks in Chapter 7 for inspiration.

Eating a whole food plant-based diet is literally like giving your internal body a bath. I found it totally cleansed my system. This is why although you may choose a gradual transformation, you should never forget that you're working towards an end goal. Moreover, remind yourself that the end goal comes with countless benefits. Optimum health and fitness, the loss of unhealthy weight, clearer skin, more focus and much more mental clarity. The list goes on.

It's time to prioritize your health and the start of a beautiful new relationship with food. Just like any relationship, if you're mindful, kind, compassionate and loving, the result will be a happier and healthier you.

Chapter 6

Time to Train: The Fit Vegan Workout

Regular exercise is, I believe, as essential as healthy eating when it comes to our quality of life and wellbeing. Getting your heart rate up regularly and using your muscles is something we all need to do as humans if we want to live a healthy life.

My 12-week Fit Vegan Workout Plan (*see Appendix, pp.219–228*) is suitable for people of all levels of fitness. There are beginner, intermediate and advanced options that you can use either at home or in the gym, and I'll tell you how to ensure the workout is pitched for your body. Built into my programme is the potential for each exercise in this chapter to be scaled up as you progress – by increasing the weights you use, the number of sets you perform and the circuits you pick as you get stronger and fitter.

But before we get into the specifics, let's talk a little bit about the calorie-maths that underlies my recommendations. At a basic level, if you're going to maintain a healthy weight, you need to make sure your calorie intake is matched by your activity level. And if your goal is to lose weight, you have to burn more calories than you consume. Only you know whether your focus needs to be on weight loss, fat loss (and muscle gain), or maintenance, but it's essential to be clear with yourself about this, and do some calculations to work out roughly what you should be burning in your workouts and consuming in your meals.

The complicated bit is knowing your precise burn rate (the speed that your body burns calories or, more accurately, glucose). In fact, it's easy to calculate your BMR (basal metabolic rate) and also your TDEE (total daily energy expenditure) – see opposite for information about these calculations. The difference between these two figures will tell you whether you have a deficit or a surplus of calories, and whether, as a result, you're likely to lose weight, maintain your current weight or gain weight. This figure will tell you what you need to adjust.

Think about it like this: if you consume 2,500 calories a day but you're only burning 2,000 calories (your TDEE), what do you think happens to the remaining 500 that you haven't used up? That's right, they don't just disappear. If only! The potential energy your body doesn't expel will ultimately get stored as fat. On the flip side, being in a slight calorie deficit every day will chip away at your fat store. I always recommend a 250–500-calorie deficit for clients with weight-loss goals. Not abiding by this rule is the simple reason why a lot of people struggle to lose weight, regardless of how hard they're training or even how healthily they're eating. A calorie is a calorie whether you're getting it from veg or chocolate. If you consume more calories than you burn, the excess will get stored as fat. Simple maths!

Key calculations

BMR (basal metabolic rate): the number of calories the body burns while at rest (assuming it isn't in the process of digesting and absorbing food).

TDEE (total daily energy expenditure): this is your BMR plus the amount of energy you burn through physical activity (not just 'formal' exercise), and the thermic effect of the food you eat. In other words, the energy your body uses up breaking down the macronutrients into the amino acids, sugars and fatty acids it needs for fuel.

NEAT (non-exercise activity thermogenesis): this is the official term for the energy you use in activity. My NEAT plays a huge role in my TDEE as I'm always super active, whether running or cycling to most places, or playing tag with my daughter. In contrast to that, an office worker who sits at a desk for eight hours a day will have a lower NEAT.

Working out your BMR

You can work out your BMR (basal metabolic rate) using the Harris-Benedict equation. This calorie formula uses your age, weight, height and sex to determine your BMR. The formula, however, doesn't take into account your lean body mass and so results in an underestimated caloric need if you're extremely muscular and an overestimated caloric if you're extremely overweight.

Men:

BMR = 66 + (13.7 × weight in kg)
        + (5 × height in cm) – (6.8 × age)

Women:

BMR = 655 + (9.6 × weight in kg)
        + (1.8 × height in cm) – (4.7 × age)

Let me use the above formula with my statistics to calculate my BMR quickly to show you what I mean:

BMR = 66 + (13.7 × 94kg = 1,288)
        + (5 × 177cm = 885) – (6.8 × 35 = 238)

BMR = 66 + 1,288 + 885 – 238

BMR = 2,001

This is the number of calories my body requires to stay alive. Now that I have my BMR, I can calculate my TDEE (total Daily

Energy Expenditure) simply by multiplying my BMR using the following activity multiplier:

Activity multiplier		
Sedentary	BMR × 1.2	(little to no exercise, desk job)
Lightly active	BMR × 1.375	(little exercise/sports 1–3 days/week)
Moderately active	BMR × 1.55	(moderate exercise/sports 3–5 days/week)
Very active	BMR × 1.725	(hard exercise/sports 6–7 days/week)
Extra active	BMR × 1.9	(hard daily exercise/sports and physical job)

With a BMR of 2001, I multiply that number by 1.725 (my current activity level of 'very active') to get a TDEE of 3,451 calories. I try not to go over 2,401 calories on non-training/sedentary days, which helps maintain my weight. Consuming less than your TDEE a day is something I simply wouldn't advise. I always go by the motto, 'Give your body what it needs,' and mine needs 2,401 (2001 × 1.2) on a sedentary day. I don't have many sedentary days, and my exercise regime is quite rigorous, burning 500–1,000 calories per day. So, for me to be at a calorie deficit of 500, I consume 1,901 calories on sedentary days and 2,951 calories on my super active days.

Working out your TDEE

When it comes to calculating your TDEE (Total Daily Energy Expenditure), you can also use an online calculator and input the required statistics. Just Google TDEE and you'll find many options to choose from. Once again, this will tell you roughly how many calories you should be consuming a day, depending on how active you are. You can then just minus 500 to be in that deficit.

A word of warning though, if you overestimate how active you are, it's easy to be off with your calculations. This is something I've seen on numerous occasions with friends questioning why they haven't met their target weight despite doing the calculations. For this reason, I recommend wearing a smartwatch that will give you an indication of how many calories you're burning daily.

My fitness journey

Now we're done with the number crunching, let's get back to talking about exercise. I've always loved being active. Football was my first love. When visiting family in Paris in the summer holidays as a child, I'd spend most of my days with my older brother playing football in the park with the other kids. I always played in my school team and was a member of a local team as well. I loved everything about the sport except watching it, as all that would do is make me want to play. I've never been one for sitting down in one place for too long, and in my teens, I began to get interested in fitness. At first, I'll be honest, I was motivated by gaining muscle. I found from doing a few press-ups on occasion that I gained muscle reasonably quickly, but I had no initial interest in the gym. I liked playing football and certainly wasn't interested in bodybuilding.

After a trip to visit my cousins in the USA, I had a change of heart when I was introduced to the gym. My cousin Benedict trained every day and encouraged me to work out, teaching me the correct techniques and several split body routines. Over the four week summer holiday, he helped me progress to a stage at which I was performing three sets of 10 repetitions of each exercise and was able to benchpress 80kg (175lb). That seems insignificant now, but understand that four weeks previously I could barely perform five reps with 60kg (130lb). This clearly demonstrated to me that I could change the way I looked and felt, as well as improve my physical strength and performance. I was always happy with the way I looked – I was a slim boy with reasonable definition – but after just four weeks of training six to seven times a week, 60–75 minutes a day, there was a noticeable change. My body responded really, really well. Not only that but my strength dramatically increased. Training and hard work really pay off, but you have to want it. I was fast becoming addicted to the feeling of being strong, fit and healthy, and I loved it.

Exercise has got me through numerous challenges in my life. The gym was always somewhere I could work off my frustrations and escape from stress. After my mother died, it was my gym routine that kept me focused. It strengthened my body, but it gave me mental clarity too. It gave me an outlet to a degree, for my sadness and frustration. It felt like a release when I worked out, and in retrospect, I think it saved me from falling into a deep depression. But as the years went by, I began to find my workouts boring and started to resent the fact I needed to spend so much time in the gym to maintain my fitness. It felt as if there was a shift in fitness culture too: the gym suddenly felt superficial and less welcoming.

The types of people I saw in the gym changed. A younger crowd began to emerge, and the steroid culture was expanding fast. Young men who didn't want to put the time in instead turned to steroids for quick results. People seemed to be more obsessed with the way they looked rather than coming to the gym to have a great workout.

Then, a year ago, I discovered CrossFit. A few friends had tried to introduce this training method to me, but I wasn't interested. I was a creature of habit, and I didn't understand what was so different about this approach to training. But since I've started training with a local CrossFit club, I've rediscovered my love of exercise. I love the diversity of the training, and the fact it takes a holistic approach. It's also incredibly inclusive; there are elderly people and teenagers alongside gym regulars like me. I love that. Now, doing a mixture of high-intensity training, I work on my cardio and respiratory endurance, strength, stamina, flexibility, power, speed, agility, balance, mobility, coordination and accuracy. The workouts are varied, and the fitness gains have been impressive.

Inspired by this, I've decided to apply the same principles of the fitness circuit to my 12-week plan. All the moves are designed to give you a full-body workout, and many of them are 'compound' exercises which means you work out more than one muscle group at once – think of it as a double-duty workout!

Many of the exercises in my workout programme are based around functional movements that mimic the way we use our body in everyday life (the antithesis of the traditional barbell shoulder press that comes to mind when I think back to my bodybuilding days). For example, the air squat in my programme mimics bending down to pick up an object from the floor.

The stop-start interval and rest nature of the workouts in this book will help keep you focused. It's easier to give 100 per cent when you know rest is around the corner. Having said that, repeated high-intensity intervals in the workouts (they'll get you sweaty, fast), maximize the afterburn effect, ensuring your body continues to burn calories even long after you've finished exercising.

First, I'll take you through my 12-week fitness programme, which is designed for all levels of fitness and can be performed in the comfort of your own home, out in the park, or even in the gym if you so wish.

High-intensity interval training (HIIT)

You'll notice with this workout programme that there's no 'steady state' cardio. I'm not asking you to spend 60 minutes on a treadmill or an exercise bike. That isn't because it's a waste of time; I really recommend incorporating some cardio into your week because it's a great mood booster and a brilliant way to increase your BMR. It's also an easy way to try out high-intensity interval training (HIIT) as you can intersperse intervals of slow-paced jogging with sprints (or for beginners, walking with jogging).

HIIT benefits

The workouts in my programme focus on resistance exercises (although some, such as burpees and bear crawls, are very dynamic). The stop-start nature of this workout is all part of the plan. It turns the workout into HIIT training, which gives the maximum afterburn effect. This ensures your body continues to burn energy after you've finished your workout. Now that's what I call a result! Sounds too good to be true, right? The body continues to use energy after HIIT workouts to aid recovery and help us cool down, as well as dealing with hormonal changes that specific exercises cause in our body. It's for this reason that HIIT is a must if your goal is weight loss. Even if it isn't, there are so many other benefits. I'm yet to hear a client complain about burning calories while chilling on the sofa or lying down.

Workout equipment

If you plan to work out at home rather than in a gym, you'll need to invest in the following equipment. You don't need to spend a fortune, and you can often pick up equipment second-hand. The money this will save on gym membership and the time you'll save not travelling to and from the gym will undoubtedly make this kit one of the best investments you can make.

- Dumbbells × 2: 8–16kg for women; 16–24kg max for men
- Kettlebell × 1: 8–16kg for women; 16–24kg max for men
- Pull-up bar × 1: You can buy these online to fit the inside of a doorframe
- Skipping rope × 1
- TRX straps
- Yoga mat

This programme will take you from your current fitness level (whether that's sedentary or already pretty fit) to being in the best condition you've ever experienced.

Warm-up and post-workout stretching

Warming up and stretching before and after you've worked out is of paramount importance. It might feel like a waste of time, but by warming up before you exercise, and stretching correctly afterwards, you're safeguarding yourself from injury and reducing your risk of DOMS (delayed onset muscle soreness), that horrible feeling where you ache terribly days after you've worked out. By warming up properly, what you're effectively doing is preparing your body for the strenuous task it's about to complete. A warm-up needs to be tailored to match the type of workout you're doing too. It isn't a one-size-fits-all thing. The great thing about my programmes is that they contain all the components of fitness. It's because of this that we also have to incorporate all body systems in the warm-up. This includes your cardiovascular (heart, lungs and respiratory system), as well as your muscle and nerve pathways (neuromuscular systems), and the joints (skeletal system).

By warming up, you allow your body systems to adjust gradually as you steadily raise your pulse rate, increasing your body's temperature. Similarly, stretching helps to lengthen muscles, providing a more effective range of motion again reducing the risk of injury. At the same time as limbering up, or stretching your muscles, a proper warm-up or cool-down should simultaneously mobilize the joints with the release of synovial fluid. This reduces the risk of soft tissue injury and also reduces lactic acid build-up in the early stages of training.

Here are three more reasons to warm up properly:

- Your blood vessels widen, increasing the blood flow to your heart and the delivery of oxygen to your muscles.

- Metabolic activity in the muscle is stimulated, resulting in higher calorie burn.

- Your heart is better prepared to respond to more strenuous exercise if you've already raised your heart rate somewhat by warming up.

There are so many reasons that make your warm-up essential. It should be mandatory. Nothing frustrates me more than seeing PTs go straight into a session with a client with no warm-up. It really is a recipe for disaster, so please make sure you don't skip it when you're exercising on your own.

Here is my warm-up, which you might like to follow before using the Fit Vegan Workout.

WARM-UP EXERCISES

I always begin by warming the joints with 3–5 minutes of light jogging on the spot and a routine of dynamic stretches that mimic the moves I'm about to perform. You can find videos of these exercises on my YouTube channel (www.youtube.com/EdricKennedy-Macfoy) and my website (www.edrickm.com).

Alternating vertical twist × 5

Stand with your feet a little wider than shoulder width apart. Place your hands one on top of the other in front of your chest, palms facing down and parallel with the ground.

Contract the muscles in your legs and core, then alternatively twist to the left and right keeping your hips square and your head in neutral alignment with your body on each rotation.

Jumping jack × 15

Stand with your feet together while you place your hands down by your sides. Slightly bend your knees, then jump up and raise your arms above your head, jumping your legs out wide, so they land outstretched. Reverse the motion by jumping back to the starting position.

Skier jumping jack × 10

Stand in a neutral position with your right foot forward and arms by your sides. Keeping your right arm straight, swing your left arm up and forward as far as your range of motion will allow. Then jump-switch your stance, softening the knees on impact, so that your left foot is forward and the right arm is raised.

Alternating lunge with an elbow-to-ankle stretch and rotation × 4

Begin in the lunge position with your right leg forward, foot flat on the floor and a 90-degree bend at the knee. The left leg is extended behind you with either the top or ball of the foot on the floor.

Place your left palm to the floor directly beneath your left shoulder and in line with your right foot, and your right palm just inside your right foot. Keep your spine neutral.

Lift your right hand off the floor, bending the elbow 90 degrees and reaching towards the instep of your right foot. Reach as far as you can without rounding your back.

As you ascend to the starting position, rotate your torso to the right and press through the left palm as you extend your right arm to the ceiling, palm facing outwards. Keep the spine long as you continue reaching through the back leg. Repeat x 4 then repeat on other side.

Single leg side lunge × 4

Step out to the side and lunge with your knee flexing forward but not shooting over your toes. Repeat with the other leg.

Walkout × 3

Stand tall, engage your core and fold your upper body forward, putting your palms on the floor in front of you (you may need to bend your knees a little). Walk your hands out to a plank position, then back again, returning to standing.

Perform this warm-up before each workout.

***

The workout

The frequency, level of challenge and type of workout you choose will vary depending on your fitness goals, your lifestyle and your preferences.

The workout programme in the Appendix (*see pp.219–228*) can be done at home and in the gym. For those who aren't aiming to build muscle but instead want to work on their overall fitness and body conditioning, it's a super-effective full-body circuit. In addition to this, you'll find a more advanced workout plan on my website (www.edrickm.com).

In general, I'd recommend opting for a gym-based workout if your goal is to build muscle, as the targeted and incremental increase in weights is the best way to achieve hypertrophy (growth in muscle mass).

The workout has options for varying levels of fitness, so pick the level that best suits you and build from there. For beginners, aim for at least three workouts per week, and be sure to allow for a full day's rest between workouts as the circuit challenges all your muscle groups in one go. More advanced fitness enthusiasts will be able to cope with daily workouts, but it's a good idea to avoid overly fatiguing the same muscle groups two days in a row however fit you are.

I can't be more prescriptive than this because what works for one person could be too much or too little for the next. Just be realistic about what is achievable and will work for you.

Choosing the right weights

The first thing to remember when choosing weights is that whether you're a total beginner or an accomplished athlete, it's a good idea to know your 1 rep max (1RM). This can support your training as you move towards achieving your goals.

Your 1RM is the maximum weight your body can lift for 1 repetition and is an indicator of your muscular strength. In the UK there's an estimated 1RM guide that sets out the percentages per rep following 100 per cent at one rep.

So, if 100kg was my 1RM for a bench press, that would be 100 per cent at 1 rep. At 2 reps my max would be 95kg, (95 per cent of my 1 rep max), 3 reps would be 93kg (93 per cent of my 1 rep max); 4 reps 90kg (90 per cent of my 1 rep max), and so on. See The Fit Vegan Workout Plan in the Appendix (*see pp.219–228*) for the numbers of reps per exercise and work out your 1RM for each.

An advanced lifter will already know their 1RM. Beginner and intermediate lifters can avoid overtraining and unconsciously working against their goals by working out their 1RM and different rep ranges according to their goal of strength, endurance or hypertrophy.

For a beginner, I recommend finding a weight that you can perform no more than the number of reps you're aiming for. In other words, if you're performing four sets of 8 reps, you'd want to select a weight that you can do 8 reps of, struggle to get 9 and definitely can't complete 10. It might take a bit of time and testing out when you begin, but the investment is worth it to make sure you get maximum results from your workout. Picking weights that are too light is a common problem and means you won't see the results you're hoping for.

The Fit Vegan workout moves

On the following pages I explain how to perform each of the exercises in the workout plan in the Appendix (*see pp.219–228*). The exercises are listed in A–Z order for ease of reference, and you can find a short video of each exercise on my YouTube channel (www.youtube.com/EdricKennedy-Macfoy) and my website (www.edrickm.com). The workout plan is a structured 12-week programme with three or four different workouts per week to give you a dynamic full-body workout. It has beginner, intermediate and advanced levels, so there will be something suitable whether you're just starting out at home or are already a regular gym goer who works out with weights.

AIR SQUAT

Keep your knees shoulder-width apart and in line with your toes throughout this exercise.

1. Step your feet to just wider than shoulder-width apart.

2. Squat down as far as you can. Your hips should be lower than your knees if you're able.

3. Maintain the lumbar curve in your spine, keeping it neutral, and keep your heels on the floor, letting your weight move into your heels.

4. Push back up to standing through your heels, standing tall at the top of the squat.

ALTERNATE LUNGE

1. Stand tall with your feet hip-width apart.

2. Step forward with your right leg, and, keeping your spine in neutral alignment, lower your body until you create a 90-degree bend at the front knee joint. Your left knee should be hovering lightly above the floor.

3. Return to the starting position and repeat with the other leg.

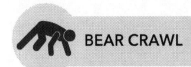

BEAR CRAWL

A bear crawl can be done with minimal space, i.e. using the length of a yoga mat or a cleared space in your home. In the gym, you could use the warm-up space or mat area.

1. Start in a press-up position with the hands shoulder-width apart and legs straight out directly behind your body, hip-width apart. Keep your knees bent.

2. Push the toes of your left foot into the floor while squeezing your right thigh and glute.

3. Move your left hand and right leg forward to start crawling.

4. Alternate the arm and leg movements while keeping the back straight and the hips and shoulders at the same height. Crawl for the desired distance.

BROAD JUMP

1. Stand with your feet shoulder-width apart, arms in the air.

2. Swing your arms down in front of you and back behind your body as you bend your knees and push your hips back.

3. Swing your arms forward as you drive the feet down and push your hips forward as you propel off the ground in a forward jump.

4. Land on your feet and return to your start position.

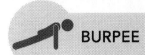

BURPEE

1. Drop into a squat position and place your hands on the floor in front of you, shoulder-width apart, and jump your feet back to a plank position.

2. Jump your legs back to a squat, feet landing by your hands.

3. Push up through your thighs and buttocks to a standing position.

4. Jump at the top, hands raised up.

5. Return to the squat position.

DEAD HANG

1. Grip an overhead bar or rings, and hang with your feet suspended from the floor and crossed at the ankles. Keep your arms extended and both latissimus dorsi (lats) and core engaged.

2. Sustain the dead hang hold for as long as possible without losing any core strength. Once you start to wobble, it's time to drop back down.

Dead hang: supported

This variation uses rings instead of an overhead bar for added stability and is recommended for beginners.

1. Adopt the ring row position (*see p.127*) as low as possible, and dead hang with both core and lats engaged.

2. Sustain the hold for as long as possible without losing core strength. Once you start to wobble, pull back up to a standing position and release the rings.

DIP

You'll need a chair or an exercise bench for this exercise. Sit on the edge of a sturdy bench or chair and place your hands either side of your hips. Use the added height of two chairs or exercise benches if you want to increase the intensity.

1. Make sure your fingers are gripping the edge of the surface and your palm is planted firmly.

2. Inch forward with your feet so that your hips come off the bench. Your knees should form a 90-degree angle, and your thighs should be parallel to the floor. Be sure to keep your shoulders back and down.

3. Tighten your abs and slowly lower yourself using your arms, bending your elbows, feeling your triceps working. Keep your elbows in.

4. Slowly push yourself back up to the starting position, squeezing your triceps muscles at the top of the movement.

FRONT SUPPORT HOLD

This exercise is similar to a press-up, but you hold the upper position rather than lowering to the floor.

1. Place your palms on the floor, shoulder-width apart, supporting the front of your body. Your wrists are directly beneath your shoulders, your arms are straight with elbows locked and your heels are stretching back. Your ears, shoulders, hips and ankles should be in alignment, and your glutes should be engaged.

2. Hold the position for the time specified in the workout plan.

HANDSTAND

1. Face away from the wall with your body in the front support position (*see opposite*). Distributing your weight through both hands, fingers and thumbs, walk your legs as high up the wall as is comfortable, the furthest point being the handstand position. Alternatively, kick up facing the wall.

2. Keeping your shoulders active, push into the ground.

3. Engage your core. Your body should be almost straight and as close to the wall as possible, without touching.

4. Squeeze your glutes and keep your whole body tight.

5. Extend through your heels to the ceiling.

6. To release and return to an upright position, wall walk or kick your legs back down to the floor.

HIGH KNEES (RUNNING IN PLACE)

1. Stand straight with your feet hip-width apart, arms by your sides, and look straight ahead.

2. Drive your right knee towards your chest and quickly place it back on the ground.

3. Follow immediately by driving your left knee towards your chest.

4. Continue alternating your knees as quickly as you can. Your arms should follow the motion, elbows engaged as you pump them in time with your legs.

KETTLEBELL DEADLIFT

1. Start by positioning your feet shoulder-width apart and gripping a kettlebell in each hand, on the mat, just outside your hips. Maintain the lumbar curve in your spine, with your shoulders slightly in front of your kettlebells.

2. Raise your hips and shoulders as you lift the kettlebells off the floor, keeping your weight in your heels.

3. Raise both kettlebells in a straight line following the midline of your foot.

4. At the top of the deadlift, stand up straight.

5. Keeping your core engaged and maintaining a neutral spine as you descend, return the kettlebells to the starting position just outside the hips.

KETTLEBELL SWING

1. Stand with your legs shoulder-width apart (or slightly wider).

2. Hold the kettlebell with both hands, so it's hanging down in front of your pelvis.

3. Squat down, making sure your knees don't go over your toes, maintaining the lumbar curve. Your hips descend back and down but not going over your knees.

4. As you push up, using your lower body to power you back to standing, drive the kettlebell up in an arc straight out in front of you and up, overhead, until your arms are fully extended.

5. Keep your arms straight throughout the movement as the kettlebell pendulums up from above your feet to above your head.

6. Lower your hips back to a partial squat as the kettlebell descends, ready to start your next rep.

KETTLEBELL/DUMBBELL THRUSTER

1. Begin with your feet positioned slightly wider than shoulder-width apart.

2. Hold the kettlebell with a neutral grip and in the 'racked position' (wrists straight, knuckles facing the ceiling).

3. Squat down to the appropriate depth (thighs parallel to the ground).

4. Now, explosively stand up while pushing the kettlebell directly overhead, moving the weight up your body and straight over your shoulders.

5. Take note of your finishing position. Your ankles, knees and hips should be locked out.

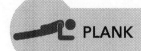 **PLANK**

Keep your legs straight with only the balls of your feet on the floor or scale by putting your thighs on the floor in a half-plank position (*see below*). This position can be scaled further by placing your knees on the mat or by performing the press-up while standing and pushing against a wall.

1. Adopt the press-up position with your legs straight and weight resting on the balls of your feet and your elbows. Your hands should be locked together on the mat in front of you.

2. Maintaining neutral alignment with your back and hips aligned, contract/tense your abdominals and pull the floor towards you.

3. Make sure your glutes are engaged throughout the hold.

Half plank

You will be able to build up to hold a half plank for longer as your fitness increases.

1. Get into a press-up position with your forearms on the floor instead of your hands.

2. Squeeze your glutes and engage your core, pulling your belly in towards your spine.

3. Create a strong, straight line from head to heels; your spine should be neutral.

4. Hold, ensuring your core, rather than your lower back, is doing the work.

Half plank knees down

As for the half plank, but your knees remain on the mat to provide additional support. This is a good options for beginners.

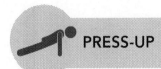

PRESS-UP

1. Place your hands on the floor, shoulder-width apart.

2. Keep your legs straight with only the balls of your feet on the floor, or scale by putting your thighs on the floor in a half-plank position (*see p.122*). This position can be scaled further by placing your knees on the mat or by performing the press-up while standing and pushing against a wall.

3. Begin in the press-up start position with your arms extended.

4. Lower your chest, hips and thighs to the floor, keeping your body rigid and your core engaged. Your elbows should be tight to your body and should point towards your hips.

5. Push the floor away and complete a full arm extension back to the start position.

Incline press-up

This is a beginner's variation of the press-up in which you place your hands on a stable chair or bench to reduce the amount of body weight you're lifting. The higher the incline, the easier the exercise will be to complete. You could also place your knees on the mat.

1. Using a bench or another stable surface, select an inclination suitable for your strength.

2. Place your hands on the surface, a little wider than shoulder-width apart.

3. With your feet fixed on the floor, bend your arms and lower your body until your chest touches the bench/surface.

4. Push your body back up to the starting position to complete the repetition.

PULL-UP

1. Jump up so that your hands grip the overhead bar, slightly wider than shoulder-width apart.

2. To begin, hang from the bar with your arms fully extended and your knees bent.

3. Engage your core and slowly pull upwards until your chin comes over the bar. Keep your chest proud but not arching to the bar.

4. Slowly move downwards until your arms are extended again to complete one pull-up.

If pull-ups can't be performed, then jumping pull-ups (jumping to get your chin over the bar and then controlling the descent), or ring rows (*see opposite*), can be effective scaling options.

RING ROW

This exercise can also be a scaled option or progression for pull-ups.

1. With the TRX strap looped over a bar at head height or higher, grip the rings and lean back until your arms are straight.

2. Keep your body straight and pull your chest up towards the rings as high as you can.

3. Pause briefly at the top of the exercise and then slowly lower yourself back down to the starting position. This is one full repetition.

Ring row supported

This variation, beginning from a more upright position, is good for anyone new to ring training as the more upright you stand the easier the exercise becomes. The aim is to lean further back, decreasing the angle between your body and the mat, as you work progressively through the programme.

SINGLE-ARM FARMER'S CARRY

Throughout this exercise, maintain a relaxed and upright posture as you carry the kettlebell for the desired time/distance.

1. Start by positioning your feet shoulder-width apart and gripping a kettlebell in one hand, on the mat, just outside your hips. Maintain the lumbar curve in your spine, with your shoulders slightly in front of your kettlebells.

2. Raise your hips and shoulders as you lift the kettlebell off the floor, keeping your weight in your heels.

3. Raise the kettlebell in a straight line following the midline of your foot.

4. At the top of the deadlift, stand up straight, engage your core and pull your ribcage down, rolling your shoulders back and down without forcing them.

5. Pull your shoulder blades in towards your spine, freeing your neck.

6. Stride for 40–50m (130–160ft), maintaining a neutral spine with your core engaged.

SINGLE-ARM KETTLEBELL HOLD

1. Stand with your feet under your hips, creating a solid base.

2. Grip a kettlebell in one hand, knuckles facing forward.

3. Engage your core and, keeping your elbow bent, lift the kettlebell to the 'racked position' (wrists straight, knuckles facing the ceiling), at shoulder height. Then drive your arm up into full extension, pointing straight up above your head.

4. Squeeze your glutes and pull your ribcage down, creating a solid midline.

5. Position the kettlebell over the centre of your body and hold still with your arm fully extended.

6. Swing the kettlebell straight down with control, using your core to stabilize yourself.

7. Return to your starting position.

SIT-UP

1. Lie on your back with your knees bent and your feet flat on the floor.

2. Place your fingertips behind your ears.

3. Pull your shoulder blades in towards your spine, so your elbows are out to the side.

4. Engage your core, then raise your upper torso towards your knees, shoulders lifting off the floor, feeling a contraction in your abs.

5. Keep your head looking straight between your knees. Don't drop your chin or pull your head forward.

6. Roll back down to the starting position.

Sit-up (advanced)

If you want to increase your workout, use this more advanced technique. Use a rolled towel or an ab mat to fill the space between the lumbar curve in your lower back and the floor or mat.

1. Begin with the soles of your feet together.

2. Reach your hands back out behind you, touching the floor at the beginning of the movement.

3. Shoot your arms forward, flexing your abdominals and pulling your torso up to a seated position, touching the floor in front of your feet.

4. Roll back to the start position.

STANDING KETTLEBELL HOLD

1. With the kettlebell in between your legs, place your feet a little wider than shoulder-width apart with your toes slightly pointed out.

2. Squat down and take hold of the kettlebell by the horns.

3. Stand tall and drive the kettlebell to your chest, keeping your elbows tucked in to your sides. Look up slightly when performing the squat to help keep your back in alignment. Ensure your knees do not overshoot your toes.

Kettlebell front squat

This exercise can be performed with one or two kettlebells, depending on your level of fitness.

1. Follow the steps for the standing kettlebell hold (*above*).

2. Keeping your heels in contact with the floor and your knees pushed outwards at all times, lower your body weight (as if you are sitting into a chair) until your thighs are parallel with the mat.

3. Pause in the squat position for 3 seconds, then push the floor away from you as you return to standing. Don't lean backwards.

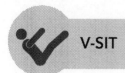

V-SIT

This is a fantastic strength-based exercise that utilizes your body weight to isolate your core. This movement will target not just your abdominals but also your back muscles, quadriceps and hamstrings.

1. Lie flat on your exercise mat in a supine (face-up) position with your legs together and straight, and your arms stretched above your head.

2. Simultaneously, raise your arms and torso, keeping them aligned, as well as your legs, until your body forms a V shape. Your chest should be open and lifted.

3. Hold for a one count (one second), then return to the starting position.

V-sit, hands by knees

1. Sit in the middle of your mat with your knees raised and the soles of your feet on the mat.

2. Lift your legs to a 45-degree angle then lean back to a 45-degree angle.

3. Reach forward with your arms activated and hovering at either side of your knees, so that you're balancing on your tailbone.

4. Hold for a one count, then return to the starting position.

V-sit, hands by thighs

1. Start in a seated position with your knees bent, arms by your side and feet off the floor. Your chest should be open and lifted.

2. Slowly unfold from your V-sit by simultaneously lowering your torso and legs towards the floor.

3. Stop when your legs reach the 45-degree angle, or if your lower back begins to arch away from the floor. Keep your head and shoulders off the floor and your lower back pressed firmly into the mat.

4. Hold for a one count, then return to the starting position.

Yoga

Yoga is an inward journey. The word yoga is derived from the Sanskrit word *yuj* which means 'union'. Yoga is the union between the individual self – the self identified with the body, mind and senses – and the universal self – the self that has been freed from all worldly limitations.

I encourage all my clients to do yoga at least once a week. This is a practice I once looked upon as something light, fluffy and for those who didn't have it in them to work out and shift some serious weights. That was before I realised the power of yoga and began practising myself. I went on to complete a 200 hour intensive yoga teacher-training course in Rishikesh, India, and have since began teaching and incorporating more yoga into my fitness regime.

Yoga, and hatha yoga in particular, provides so much more than physical benefits. It improves your physical strength, stamina and muscular endurance, but also your concentration and connection with breath through the practice of conscious breathing while practicing postures. Both your mental and emotional health benefit from a regular yoga practice. Our modern lifestyles often result in us carrying toxins in the body which result in pain, illness and stress. Yoga, in combination with the Fit Vegan regime, can help to release these toxins.

The benefits I've gained from practising yoga include:

- improved athletic performance

- increased energy

- increased flexibility

- better balance

- improved strength, stamina and muscle tone

- relief from lower back pain

- increased bone density

- stress reduction

- improved concentration

- improved immune function

- tension release from mind and body

One of the most significant benefits of regular yoga is that it helps you to become more conscious of synchronizing breath and movement. It also might help you to break the habit of holding on to breath when you're exercising. It's a useful way to retrain yourself to remember that you should breathe out at the most challenging part of any exercise when the muscle is contracting. Breathe in as you relax and recover. Breathing correctly is so important in any exercise circuit. When you move with your breath, you're so much more efficient. Breathing correctly helps you get into a good rhythm, and when you breathe out with each exertion, movements feel easier. Poor breathing habits can cause you to run out of steam long before the end of your workout, so it's worth focusing on it.

YOGA CIRCUIT

Try this quick wake-up circuit to improve mobility and circulation first thing. You can find videos of these exercises on my YouTube channel (www.youtube.com/EdricKennedy-Macfoy) and my website (www.edrickm.com).

Child's pose

1. Kneeling on your mat, fold forward over your knees, bringing your forehead to the ground in front of you.

2. Stretch your arms out along the mat in front of you, enjoying the feeling of release and opening in your hips, shoulders and back.

3. Hold for a minute, breathing deeply and fully.

4. For an extra back-opener, walk both hands to one side of the mat, feeling the lateral stretch down your side. Make sure you do this to both sides.

Downward-facing dog

1. From child's pose, push up on to all fours.

2. Taking your weight into your toes, lift your knees, pushing your bottom up and back as you exhale.

3. Raise your hips until your arms are straight.

4. Pedal through your feet, dropping your heels to the ground one by one and stretching the backs of your legs. Exhale on each 'effort'.

5. Keep your knees bent if it feels like a strain to straighten your legs fully.

6. Hold for a minute, then release back to child's pose.

Cat-cow

1. Get into an all-fours position on your hands and knees.

2. Exhale as you round your spine, like a cat, neck stretching downwards, and tail down.

3. Extend your arms fully as you let your spine curve and stretch.

4. Reverse the motion for cow: as you inhale, curve your spine the opposite way as you lift your tailbone and arch your back, shoulders pulling together on your spine as your head and neck lift.

5. Transition from cat to cow fluidly every few seconds for a minute, mobilizing your spine.

Yoga lunge

1. From a standing position, lunge backwards with your right leg, exhaling as you lower your right knee until it's hovering a few inches above the floor.

2. Raise your arms above your head, pulling your shoulder blades together on your back and allowing your neck to feel free. Your left knee should be aligned over your left heel.

3. Engage your core as you hold the position, breathing fluidly.

4. Hold for 20 seconds, then return to your starting position and repeat on the other side.

You get out what you put in

I'm a firm believer in what you put in is what you get out. Listen to your body and remember this is your journey, your growth and your development. Just like veganism, try not to run before you can walk. The aim is to push your body to its limit while remaining injury-free. Warming up, cooling down and practising yoga will help you to support your body to recover from your workouts.

Share your journey with me at www.edrickm.com. I'd love to hear about your progress and find out how you get on with my programmes.

Chapter 7

Fit Vegan Meals and the Vegan-Ready Kitchen

The recipes in this chapter are designed to be easy and quick to make, delicious, nutritious and portion-controlled. They are also balanced, providing you with the right ratio of protein, carbs and fats. I've based them all around plant-based whole foods, with the emphasis on easy-to-source ingredients you'll be able to find in most supermarkets. All of these recipes have been tried and tested by me, and I give you my word that they're tasty and filling.

Although this isn't a 'diet' in the traditional sense of the word, I've kept the calorie count at a healthy level, mindful of the BMR (basic metabolic rate) and TDEE (total daily energy expenditure) ratios we discussed in the previous chapter (*see p.93*). I've given you five options for breakfast, lunch and dinner, and there are also suggested snacks to keep you going pre- and post-workout. Do check out my YouTube channel (www.youtube.com/EdricKennedy-Macfoy) if you're keen to get extra inspiration.

Finally, I'll reveal how to get your kitchen vegan-ready, with store-cupboard staples to stock up on and versatile ingredients to keep in your fridge for those times when you need something quick and nutritious.

Breakfast

I think it's important to clarify precisely what breakfast is. If you look in the dictionary, you'll find breakfast to be 'a meal eaten in the morning, the first of the day'. But like most things, I have my own definition and call it 'break fast'. Breakfast is simply that – the time when you eat your first meal, breaking your fast, whether it's 6 a.m. or 12 p.m.

So, where did the notion that breakfast is the most important meal of the day come from? Before a little research, my answer to that question would've been, 'My mum,' because that's what she used to say. But after researching the evidence for the statement, I came up short. John Kellogg, the cereal tycoon, was the first to coin the phrase – one that served his interests for obvious reasons!

At one time, I used to eat breakfast within an hour of waking in the morning; it was what my body was used to, and I'd come to think of it as healthy. Now, after trying intermittent fasting a few times, I break my fast at 12 p.m. most days. However, if I'm training in the morning, I find my performance is always better if I've fuelled my body with an adequate pre-workout meal. If I'm training later in the day, delaying breakfast till noon isn't an issue.

I always advise my clients to listen to their body. Are you hungry first thing in the morning? How are your energy levels? Test your performance with and without breakfast and see where you stand. I think as long as you're getting all the nutrients your body needs daily, whether or not you choose to eat breakfast (and indeed when you choose to eat it) is irrelevant. Listen to your body. The more important question is, what do you have for breakfast?

I always find the food I choose to break my fast makes all the difference to my day. However, I start every day by drinking a glass of warm lemon water, turmeric and black pepper before eating anything. This simple beverage has countless health benefits, but like everything I eat, the proof is in the pudding. This concoction transformed my mornings which, if I'm honest, were already pretty amazing. So, if you don't know, I'm about to let you know why I break my fast with lemon and turmeric water every single day.

I'm going to start with lemons because they equal my favourite word – energy. I've always been very energetic, especially first thing in the morning, so I was surprised that I even noticed an increase in my energy levels. Although lemons are acidic, introduce them to your body and they have an alkalizing effect. That being said, the acid can damage tooth enamel, and dentists advise waiting for 20 minutes after eating lemons before brushing your teeth. Drinking water alone first thing in the morning sets the tone for the day. You're hydrating yourself, which is key to good health and can also help prevent kidney issues. Not only are you upping your fluid intake, but lemons contain flavonoids, which are antioxidants and have antioxidant properties. These substances have been said to help protect your cells from damage and disease. Lemons are also extremely high in vitamin C and squeezing the juice from just half a lemon will give you around 25 per cent of your daily intake. Vitamin C is essential for the development and repair of all bodily tissues.

Changing how you break your fast is the first thing that I suggest to clients, and I'm yet to have anyone report back saying they didn't experience numerous benefits, including weight loss. If you're just going to have the lemon water alone, which some of my clients do, it doesn't really matter if the water is tepid, hot or cold. My morning beverage varies with my mood and the temperature outside. In the summer months, I squeeze the juice of several lemons into ice trays and freeze it, so I have fresh lemon juice available at any time.

As for the addition of turmeric, my older brother Adonis introduced this to me and I honestly thought it was a prank – especially when he threw in a mention of black pepper. That said, I was aware of the fact that turmeric is used as a natural medicine in many cultures and that black pepper is made from dried berries and also has several health benefits. When you mix the two together, the health benefits are multiplied. Turmeric contains a compound called curcumin which helps your body to shed fat really quickly. The problem is, our bodies struggle to absorb turmeric, but that's where the black pepper comes in. It boosts the bioavailability by 2,000 per cent.

Lemon water is a healthy alternative to more sugary beverages that come with additional health benefits. If you don't fancy adding turmeric and black pepper to it, don't.

Until a few years ago, I ate cereal every morning. The funny thing is, I didn't even notice the effect of my poor food choices until I made some improvements and truly began to feel the difference. I noticed that my energy levels improved. I was less likely to get hungry before lunch and better able to concentrate. A healthy breakfast ensures you start the day as you mean to go on. Pack your body full of those essential nutrients and reduce the risk of succumbing to unhealthy cravings later on. Here are five great options to try.

Porridge with nuts and seeds

Serves 1

This is my go-to breakfast. Porridge is an excellent source of minerals and vitamins and also rich in zinc, copper and iron. With the addition of nuts and seeds, I'm also getting a big hit of fibre and protein. This hearty breakfast choice used to fuel my long shifts in the fire service. There were countless times when I'd be flying around on the back of the machine on the way to a fire while eating my oats and rigging for the job. This recipe is simple to customize too – just add your favourite fruit, nuts and seeds.

90g/3oz/1 cup porridge oats

½ tsp ground cinnamon

⅛ tsp sea salt

1 tsp agave syrup

1 chopped banana

240ml/16fl oz/1 cup plant milk of choice

Ideas for toppings

1 tbsp chia seeds

1 tbsp flax seeds

1 tbsp pumpkin seeds

2 tbsp goji berries

2 tbsp mixed nuts

Combine all the dry ingredients in a bowl. Top with the agave syrup and banana. Pour over the milk and top with your choice of dried nuts, seeds or berries.

Kale, date and banana nut smoothie

Serves 1

When you don't have time to sit down, this is a great option. You can pour the smoothie into a flask and go. Often, before a super-early-morning training session, I just don't feel like eating, and this is when this shake comes into play. Great for both pre- and post-workout fuel, as both dates and bananas are packed full of potassium, which makes them the perfect food to help combat post-workout muscle soreness.

3 Medjool dates, chopped and destoned

480ml/1 pint/2 cups plant milk of choice (I use almond)

2 tbsp nut butter of choice (I use almond)

2 frozen bananas

1 handful kale

Place all the ingredients in a blender and blitz until smooth. Add water for desired consistency and blend again until well combined.

Vegan breakfast wrap

Serves 1

We all get those days where we crave a hot breakfast. I used to eat sausages, bacon and eggs, which left me feeling heavy, sluggish and lethargic. But this wrap satiates me and is perfect for the morning after a big night out.

> 1 tortilla wrap
>
> 1x 200g/7oz can mixed beans, drained and rinsed
>
> 1 tbsp salsa
>
> Pinch of sea salt
>
> ½ tsp cumin
>
> ½ tsp paprika
>
> 1 tbsp olive oil
>
> 150g/5oz/2 cups oyster mushrooms, shredded
>
> 1 garlic clove, minced
>
> 1 tbsp red onion, diced
>
> Sea salt and black pepper to taste

Place a tortilla wrap on a plate, ready to fill. Throw the mixed beans in a bowl with the salsa, cumin, paprika and sea salt. Mash thoroughly and set aside.

Heat the olive oil in a large pan on a medium heat. Add the oyster mushrooms and garlic to the pan and stir fry gently until cooked.

Spoon the beans and mushrooms onto the tortilla wrap. Sprinkle the red onion over the top and season with sea salt and black pepper to taste. Gently roll up the tortilla and enjoy.

Coconut quinoa delight

Serves 2

Until recently, I thought of quinoa as a savoury ingredient, but then I visited a café where I tried quinoa porridge; it really changed my mind. Whether sweet or savoury, quinoa tastes great and it's super-nutritious. It's also low on the glycaemic index (GI) scale, meaning it digests slowly, so won't cause a rapid spike in your blood sugar levels followed by an inevitable crash. It's also a great source of protein.

90g/1oz/½ cup quinoa, cooked to packet instructions

880ml/1½ pints/3 cups coconut milk

½ tsp cinnamon

1 tbsp agave/maple syrup

1 tsp vanilla extract

2 tbsp chopped kiwi

2 tbsp chopped mango,

2 tbsp chopped pineapple,

1 tbsp chia seeds

1 tbsp flax seeds

1 tbsp sunflower seeds

Combine the quinoa, coconut milk, cinnamon, agave syrup and vanilla extract in a saucepan and cook until the quinoa can be fluffed with a fork.

Divide the quinoa between two bowls and top with kiwi, mango and pineapple. Drizzle a little coconut milk over the fruit and top with seeds. I often have this without the agave syrup as I find the fruit makes it sweet enough. You may want to try with and without.

Breakfast super bowl

Serves 4

This super bowl isn't only nutritious but also calorie-dense and absolutely delicious. Super bowls are becoming more and more common, and I often get ideas for new ingredients when visiting some of my favourite restaurants. The first meal of the day kickstarts your metabolism and has a massive impact on your energy level. The difference in satiety and energy between this option and, let's say two slices of toast and Marmite is incomparable. Start your day the right way.

1 block extra-firm tofu

1 tsp olive oil

1 garlic clove, minced

½ red onion, chopped

1 tsp Italian seasoning

½ tsp ground paprika

¼ tsp ground cumin

½ tsp ground turmeric

½ tsp sea salt

½ tsp ground black pepper

100g/3½oz/½ cup canned chickpeas, drained and rinsed

½ tsp ground cumin

½ tsp chilli powder

¼ tsp sea salt

½ tsp ground black pepper

Sriracha yoghurt

2 tbsp sriracha

150g vegan coconut yoghurt

½ tsp sea salt

½ tsp ground black pepper

Added extras

1 large avocado, halved and sliced

4 tbsp cherry tomatoes, sliced

1 handful kale, chopped

4 tbsp pine nuts

Remove the excess liquid from the tofu block. I wrap mine in kitchen paper towels and place a plate on top allowing the tissue to absorb the moisture. Heat the olive oil on a medium heat then throw in the block of tofu. Chop it up with your wooden spoon or spatula while it's cooking, then add the garlic, red onion, Italian seasoning, paprika, cumin and turmeric. Gently combine the ingredients, ensuring all the tofu is evenly coated. Cook for 10 minutes over a low heat then remove and season with salt and pepper.

Pour the chickpeas into a medium pan and cover lightly with hot water. Stir in the cumin, chilli powder, sea salt and black pepper. Combine well and continue to cook over a medium heat for 5 minutes.

To make the sriracha yoghurt, combine all the ingredients for it in a large bowl and whisk until well combined.

Place a portion of the tofu and chickpeas in a bowl. Throw in the added extras of your choice and drizzle with sriracha yoghurt to complete.

Lunch

Lunchtime! You've had a hearty breakfast, and it's kept you going through to lunch. Take care not to stumble and fall at this danger point. Don't wait for hunger to strike and give in to unhealthy cravings, especially when you're out and about, or at your desk with limited options. These quick and simple recipes will ensure you're always ready with calorie-dense and nutritious food to hand.

Apple and quinoa salad

Serves 1

This is one of my favourite salads for the simple reason that I get the perfect combination of sweet and salty. Packed with ample nutrients, this delicious dish leaves me satisfied every time.

200g/7oz/1 cup quinoa, cooked according to the packet instructions

200g/7oz/1 cup edamame beans

2 handfuls spinach, finely chopped

1 green apple, sliced

½ cucumber, sliced

1 lime, squeezed

1 tbsp olive oil

½ tsp turmeric

½ tsp paprika

4 tbsp pine nuts

Sea salt and ground black pepper to taste

Place all the ingredients except the pine nuts in a bowl and gently toss to combine. Top with pine nuts and season with salt and pepper to taste.

Vegan couscous

Serves 2

Couscous is one of my favourite grains. It's light and fluffy and quickly absorbs the flavour of other ingredients. This dish is a prime example. I love it because you can literally eat it with anything. Just like its cousin quinoa, couscous works well with sweet and savoury dishes. Where I previously ate a lot of white pasta, couscous has fast become my healthier alternative. The only benefit I gained from pasta was taste. It's so high in simple carbohydrates (the same type of carbohydrate you find in sugar, white bread and other refined foods). Couscous, on the other hand, contains selenium, which is an immune-system booster and has also been said to lower cancer risk. It's a great source of protein and so easy to prep and cook.

- 1 tbsp olive oil
- 2 onions, chopped
- 2 cloves garlic, chopped
- 2 tomatoes, chopped
- 1 red pepper, chopped
- 1 green pepper, chopped
- 1 tbsp spring onion (scallion), sliced
- 300g/10oz/4 cups oyster mushrooms, shredded
- 100g/3½oz/½ cup canned chickpeas, drained and rinsed
- 2 tsp Italian seasoning

1 tsp all-purpose seasoning

200g/7oz/2 cups couscous, cooked in vegetable stock to
the packet instructions

2 handfuls spinach

Sea salt and black pepper to taste

Fresh coriander (cilantro), chopped, to garnish

There are two ways to cook this dish:

Method one

Heat a little olive oil in a pan over a medium heat. Add the
onions, garlic, tomatoes, peppers, spring onions, oyster
mushrooms and chick peas with the seasonings and gently
pan fry until browned.

Place the couscous in a bowl and add the cooked vegetables.
Finally, add in the spinach and gently combine. Season with a
sprinkle of sea salt and pepper to taste before garnishing with
the coriander. Serve with your favourite salad.

Method two

Place the onions, garlic, tomatoes, peppers, and
600ml/1½ pints/3 cups of water in a blender and whizz until
smooth. Pour the liquid into a pan, add the chickpeas and
seasoning, and cook on a medium heat for 10 minutes.

While this is cooking, heat a little olive oil in a pan over a
medium heat and shallow fry the oyster mushrooms with a

pinch of salt and pepper (and an optional splash of white wine) until gently browned. Set aside.

Remove the vegetables and chickpeas from the heat. Add the couscous, spinach and spring onions to the pot, stir and cover with a lid. Now sit back for 10 minutes to allow the couscous to soak up the flavours. Then add in the mushrooms and seasonings, and gently combine. Season with sea salt and pepper to taste before garnishing with the coriander. Serve with your favourite salad.

Stuffed pittas

Serves 1

Previously I'd always get stuck in a rut when it came to sandwich and pitta fillings. I got tired of having the same sandwich over and over again and craved variety. With a few extra minutes of prep and a bit more thought, I began to make my pitta lunch option a whole lot more interesting. There are many ways to change up this recipe, but this is one of my favourite concoctions.

2 handfuls kale, chopped

150g/5oz/2 cups oyster mushrooms, shredded

1–2 handfuls leftover veg (e.g. peppers, tomatoes and asparagus), chopped

2 wholemeal pitta pockets

4 tbsp hummus

Heat a little olive oil in a pan over a medium heat and shallow fry the oyster mushrooms with the peppers, tomatoes and asparagus (or leftover veg) for 8–10 minutes until gently browned and cooked through. Set aside.

In a bowl, combine the cooked vegetables with the kale. Season with salt and pepper to taste.

Toast the pitta pockets, cut open and spread with the hummus, then stuff with the vegetable and mushroom mixture.

Grilled Mediterranean veg wrap

Serves 2

This is another favourite option for lunch because this hearty wrap keeps me going all afternoon, no matter how busy my schedule.

- 1 large aubergine (eggplant), thinly sliced
- 2 medium courgettes (zucchini), cut lengthwise into batons
- 2 tsp olive oil
- 2 tbsp hummus
- 2 handfuls spinach, chopped
- 2 handfuls rocket leaves
- 2 tbsp sundried tomatoes, chopped
- 2 tortilla wraps
- 4 tbsp hummus
- 2 tbsp pine nuts
- Salt and pepper to taste

Lightly coat both sides of courgette (zucchini) and aubergine slices with olive oil and add a dash of sea salt and black pepper. Place in a pan and gently fry on medium heat for about 5 minutes each side or until browned.

Spread the hummus on the wraps, and top with the courgette and aubergine slices. Add the spinach, rocket and sun-dried tomatoes, and scatter on the pine nuts. Season with salt and pepper, then fold the wrap to seal and serve.

Pea soup

Serves 2

This is one of my winter favourites but also keeps me satisfied on those days when I haven't really got a big appetite but require my nutrient quota, nonetheless. So simple to make and absolutely delicious.

500g/17½oz/3½ cups frozen peas

1 vegetable stock cube, dissolved in 480ml/1 pint/2 cups of boiling water

1 tsp smoked paprika

Pinch of smoked or ordinary chilli flakes

A squeeze of lemon juice

2 garlic cloves, crushed

1 tbsp olive oil

Sea salt and pepper

Place the frozen peas in a pan with the vegetable stock on a high heat and bring to the boil. Reduce to a simmer and cook for 6 minutes until tender. Pour the peas and liquid into a blender and add the paprika, chilli flakes, lemon juice, garlic and olive oil. Blend until smooth and season to taste with sea salt and pepper.

Dinner

Winner, winner plant-based dinner! My evening meal is often the one I look forward to the most, especially after an action-packed day. A final chance to feed my heart and nourish my soul with plant-based goodness before the day draws to an end. It's also an opportunity to get my creative juices flowing as I get my cook on and prepare a tasty work of art! I love cooking in the evening, especially for friends. It's the best way to demonstrate precisely how varied and delicious plant-based eating really is.

Nut but stew

Serves 6

This amazing West African dish is one of my winter favourites. It warms and nourishes not just my body but my soul too. It was one of my mother's signature dishes. It's super easy to make and, if you're a peanut butter lover like me, you're in for a real treat with this one.

For the coriander (cilantro) rice

500ml/1 pint/2¼ cups vegetable broth

400g/14oz/2 cups uncooked basmati brown rice

240ml/16fl oz/1 cup water

1 garlic clove, minced

¼ cup fresh lime juice

1½ tbsp olive oil

1 tsp Italian seasoning

1 tsp ground cumin

Ground black pepper to taste

Sea salt to taste

3 handfuls fresh coriander (cilantro), chopped

For the stew

- 640g No Chick Strips (or similar meat substitute), chopped
- 3 tbsp olive oil
- 4 garlic cloves, minced
- 1 tsp sea salt
- 1 tsp ground black pepper
- 2 tbsp olive oil
- 2 large onions, finely chopped
- 1 tsp ground cumin
- 2 tbsp tomato paste
- 4 tbsp organic peanut butter
- 1 large sweet potato, peeled and cut into small cubes
- 1 litre/1¾ pints/3½ cups vegetable broth
- 4 handfuls kale, stems removed, chopped
- 2 tbsp sriracha hot sauce/1 scotch bonnet pepper (optional)
- 1 tsp sea salt

To make the coriander rice, place the brown rice and vegetable broth in a pan and bring to the boil on a high heat. Stir well and cover. Reduce to a low heat and allow to simmer for 45 minutes until cooked. Remove from heat and let it stand for 5 minutes. Mix up the lime juice, garlic, olive oil, Italian seasoning and cumin in a bowl. Season with salt and pepper to taste and then drizzle the mixture evenly over the rice. Finally, add the coriander and combine.

Heat the olive oil in a large pan over a medium heat and throw in the No Chick meat substitute and cook to packet guidelines. Halfway through cooking, add half the garlic, salt and ground black pepper. Once the No Chick is evenly browned, remove it from the heat and set aside in a container or wrap in foil to preserve the heat.

Add the oil to the pan and crank the heat up to high before throwing in the onions and cooking them up for 10 minutes. Keep the onions moving in the pan. Once cooked, turn the heat back down to medium, throw in the rest of the garlic, cumin and tomato puree, and combine gently. Cook for another 5 minutes before adding the peanut butter and stirring it in. Add the sweet potato to the mix. Pour in the vegetable broth as you stir and bring to a boil for 5 minutes. Throw in the No Chick meat substitute and kale, then stir. Add the hot sauce or pepper, and the salt, and leave to cook on a low heat, occasionally stirring, for 20 minutes or until the sweet potato is cooked and tender.

For added richness, lift out the sweet potato with a slotted spoon and mash before returning to the pan. Allow to simmer on a high heat uncovered for a further 5 minutes. Serve warm with the rice and garnish with coriander and lime juice.

Butternut and cauliflower smash

Serves 1

This is a tasty, healthy alternative to mashed potatoes and creates a warm, filling quick dinner full of slow-release carbohydrates.

1 small butternut squash, peeled and chopped

300g/10½oz/2 cups cauliflower, chopped

1 small red onion, chopped

1 garlic clove, chopped

1 red pepper, chopped

220g/8oz/3 cups button mushrooms, chopped

100g/3½oz/1½ cups) canned mixed beans

1 tsp smoked paprika

1 tsp dried/fresh parsley, chopped

1 tsp basil

¼ tsp cayenne pepper

Preheat the oven to 200°C/400°F/gas mark 7 and line a baking sheet with baking parchment. Arrange the butternut squash on the prepared baking sheet and roast for 10 minutes; then add the cauliflower to it. Continue to roast for a further 20 minutes until the butternut and cauliflower are tender. Remove from the oven and set aside

Heat two tablespoons of water in a large frying pan over medium heat, add the onion and garlic, cover and cook for about 5 minutes or until tender. Add the red pepper and mushrooms and cook uncovered, stirring a further 5 minutes. Add the roasted butternut squash and cauliflower, along with the beans, spices, herbs and cayenne pepper. Cook for another 5 minutes or until thoroughly heated through.

Crush the mixture a little with a spatula and then serve.

Sunshine quinoa tabbouleh

Serves 4

This delicious recipe was originally made with bulgur wheat, but as you can tell by now, quinoa is my preferred grain. This nutritious dish is one of my summer favourites as it's light, protein-rich and packed with flavour. On top of that, it's quick and simple to make.

For the quinoa

350g/12oz/1 cup quinoa, rinsed and cooked to packet instructions

400ml/14fl oz/1¾ cups vegetable broth

½ tsp turmeric powder

½ tsp paprika

½ tsp dried basil

½ tsp salt

For the dressing

4 tbsp lemon, pulped with seeds removed

4 tbsp olive oil

½ tsp sea salt

½ tsp black pepper

1 tbsp agave syrup

For the tabbouleh

1 handful fresh basil, chopped

1 handful fresh parsley, chopped

Pinch of paprika

1 × 400g/14oz can chickpeas, drained and rinsed

2 Italian plum tomatoes, chopped

1 large avocado, sliced

1 cucumber, peeled and chopped

2 spring onions (scallions), chopped

Ground black pepper

Cook the quinoa in the vegetable broth with the turmeric and the salt in a large saucepan, as directed by the packet instructions. Drain well to remove any excess moisture, then transfer the quinoa to a large bowl and set aside to cool.

To make the dressing, place all the ingredients in a bowl and mix with a fork until well combined.

When the quinoa is cooled, add the chickpeas, fresh basil and parsley, pinch of paprika, tomatoes, spring onions, avocado and cucumber, and pour over the dressing.

Season with black pepper to taste, mix gently to combine, cover and refrigerate for at least an hour before serving.

Red Thai lentil curry with wild rice

Serves 4

This curry must be one of my favourite evening meals. Not just because I love herbs and spices, but because they're also packed with antioxidants and antibacterial properties. That's right, curries with the right ingredients are super good for you and have medicinal properties.

- 350g/12oz/1 cup red lentils, rinsed and cooked to packet instructions
- 350g/12oz/1 cup wild rice, rinsed and cooked to packet instructions
- 600ml/1½ pints/3 cups water or vegetable broth
- 2 tbsp coconut oil
- vegetable stock
- 2 garlic cloves, minced
- 2 onions, diced
- 2.5cm/½in fresh ginger, chopped
- 1 red pepper, diced
- ½ tsp turmeric
- ½ tsp cumin
- 2 tbsp red Thai curry paste
- 1 tbsp tomato puree
- 400ml/14fl oz/1¾ cups vegetable broth
- 2 handfuls fresh spinach

1 × 400g/14oz can coconut milk

2 tbsp vegan coconut yoghurt

2 tbsp fresh coriander (cilantro), chopped

Cook the wild rice and lentils as per packet instructions. While the rice and lentils are cooking, heat the coconut oil in a wok over medium heat and gently stir fry the garlic, diced onions, ginger, red pepper, turmeric and cumin for about 5 minutes. Add the cooked red lentils, Thai curry paste and tomato puree and gently stir before pouring in the broth and bring to the boil. Reduce heat, add the spinach and the coconut milk and simmer for a further 15 minutes. Serve the curry on top of the wild rice. Top with the yoghurt and a sprinkle of coriander.

Quinoa stuffed peppers

Serves 2

I previously made this dish with rice, but it wasn't long until quinoa stepped in and became my grain of choice. I eat a lot of quinoa because it has fewer calories than white rice, double the protein and 15 times fewer carbs. This stuffed pepper dish is quick and easy to prepare, and it's a great dish to serve when you're entertaining. It looks beautiful on the plate and has lots of exciting textures.

    2 large red peppers, halved lengthwise and deseeded
    1 slice sourdough toast
    110g/4oz/¼ cup quinoa, cooked to the packet instructions
    1 lemon, juiced
    2 spring onions (scallions), sliced thinly
    1 clove garlic, diced
    1 handful fresh basil, roughly chopped
    3 tbsp capers drained and rinsed.
    50g/2oz/¼ cup flaked almonds
    Ground black pepper to taste
    1 tbsp olive oil

Preheat the oven to 180°C/350°F/gas mark 5. Pop the peppers into a roasting tin, cut side up, and roast for 12 minutes until very soft.

While the red peppers are cooking, pulse the sourdough toast in a blender until it forms fine breadcrumbs. Spread the crumbs in a roasting tin, and place in the oven for about 10 minutes to dry out.

Cook the quinoa according to the packet instructions in a large pan. When cooked, take off the heat and add the lemon juice, spring onions, garlic, basil, capers and almonds to the pan. Fork through until well combined and season with black pepper to taste.

Divide the quinoa mixture between the cooked red peppers, then sprinkle the top with the breadcrumbs and a drizzle of olive oil.

Place in the oven and bake for about 10 minutes, until the breadcrumbs and quinoa are crunchy and lightly browned.

Snacks (pre- and post-workout)

Did you know that fuelling your body with the right nutrition pre- and post-workout can dramatically improve how your body benefits from your exercise regime? The right pre-workout meal or snack at the right time will fuel you with the energy your body needs to complete the most gruelling workout. Likewise, fuelling your body with a post-workout meal, using the right combination of nutrients, will help you to build and repair your muscles.

I aim to have a pre-workout snack or meal 1–3 hours before training. The times I've left it longer, there has definitely been a difference in my energy levels, which in turn affects my performance and overall results. There is one pre-workout snack I often squeeze in up to 15 minutes before a session, and that's a beloved banana. They are so easy to digest, give me a big burst of energy, and are filled with antioxidants and potassium. They also help prevent cramps, something I suffer from a lot.

When it comes to fuelling after a workout, the sooner, the better. You've just put your body through its paces and expended a lot of energy. That needs to be replaced pronto with carbs, our body's preferred energy source, and protein, which provides the building blocks of muscle. For clients who are specifically looking to build muscle, I usually advise them to get a post-workout meal in the '20-minute window' after a workout for maximum benefit. If you're just maintaining your existing body shape, then eating within the hour will suffice. Making a habit of not fuelling post-workout will seriously compromise your fitness goals. I always remind clients that nutrition is the more significant piece of the puzzle. There's absolutely no point in putting 100 per cent effort into your training but only 10 per cent effort into your nutrition. It's counterproductive and makes no sense. So, if you don't want to be left feeling tired, cranky and lethargic after your workout, you know what to do.

Date, cacao and coconut energy balls

Makes 15

This is a tasty and healthy snack you can make in advance and freeze. I make a big batch every month to keep me energized – they keep really well and have become my lifesaver. I keep them on hand for a quick pre-workout bite. They taste so good; even my daughter is obsessed. You can freeze these bad boys for up to one month and keep them in the fridge for up to a week.

> 200g/7oz/2 cups ground almonds
> 400g/14oz/1 cup Medjool dates, destoned and chopped
> 4 tbsp raw cacao powder
> 1 tbsp chia seeds
> 2½ tbsp almond butter
> 2 heaped tbsp coconut oil
> 100g/4oz/1 cup desiccated coconut

Put the dates into a medium bowl and soak in water for an hour. Add the water.

Place the ground almonds, almond butter, dates, cacao powder, desiccated coconut (reserving enough to coat the finished balls) and chia seeds in a blender or food processor and whizz until smooth. If the mixture seems too thick, add a little water and blend again. Transfer the mix to a bowl and allow 30 mins for the chia seeds to soften.

Divide the mixture into 15 equal portions and roll each one into a ball using your hands.

Place the remaining coconut in a shallow dish, throw the balls in and shake them up to coat.

Trail mix

Makes 8 servings

The great thing about this lightweight, portable snack is that not only is it full of energy, but you can customize it according to your own taste. Nuts, dry fruit, dark chocolate. Choose your favourite combination. Or you can simply use mine. It's very easy to overeat on the trail mix so take care not to have more than a couple of tablespoons at a time.

115g/4oz/¾ cup cashews

115g/4oz/¾ cup salted almonds

115g/4oz/¾ cup dried cranberries

115g/4oz/¾ cup walnuts

115g/4oz/¾ cup dark chocolate, cut into small chunks.

Combine all the ingredients in a bowl until well mixed. Store in an airtight container.

Sesame bars

Makes 10 servings

Another healthy treat packed with nutrition and ample flavour. These will keep in the fridge for up to a week, but they've never lasted that long in my fridge. Great post-workout snack to replenish that energy.

50g/2oz/¼ cup prunes, pitted

50g/2oz/¼ cup dates, pitted

1 banana, peeled

1 tbsp coconut oil

1 tbsp ground cinnamon

2 tbsp agave syrup

50g/2oz/⅓ cup almonds

140g/5oz/1 cup large oats

50g/2oz/¼ cup sunflower seeds

50g/2oz/⅓ cup big juicy raisins

50g/2oz/¼ cup sesame seeds

Place all the ingredients except the sesame seeds in a blender or food processor and blitz for a few moments until a dough is formed. Press the mixture into a flat baking tray, sprinkle sesame seeds on top and refrigerate. Cut into bars and store in an airtight container.

Tamari nuts and seeds

Makes 8 servings

I really don't know if I'd have survived my first few months of veganism without these tasty nuts and seeds at hand. Similar to the trail mix, these are guilt-free in the right quantities and provide essential omega oils as well as protein, fibre and minerals. Eat them solo or toss them in a salad or curry; your taste buds won't be disappointed!

50g/2oz/¼ cup sunflower seeds

100g/4oz/⅔ cup almonds

50g/2oz/¼ cup pumpkin seeds

100g/4oz/⅔ cup cashews

1 tsp olive oil

2 tbsp tamari

1 tbsp chilli flakes

Preheat the oven to 180°C/350°F/gas mark 5.

Place the nuts and seeds in a bowl and stir through the tamari and chilli flakes. Spread the mixture on a baking tray lined with greaseproof paper, place in the oven and bake for 10 minutes or until golden brown.

Remove from the oven, and once cool place in a sealed glass storage jar.

Quick rice cakes

Serves 1 (3 rice cakes)

The great thing about rice cakes is that they're a good source of manganese, which has strong antioxidant properties and increases your bone health along with so many other benefits. The super-light snack goes pretty well with both sweet and savoury, is low in calories and fat-free. My favourite is Kallo organic wholegrain lightly salted rice cakes.

Savoury toppings

- ¼ smashed avocado topped with a spoonful of the tamari nuts and seeds mix (*see p.182*) or chilli flakes, or
- 1 tbsp oat crème fraiche, or
- 1 tbsp tahini topped with sliced tomatoes and coriander (cilantro)

Suggested sweet toppings

- 1 tbsp peanut butter, or
- ½ banana, chopped, or
- ½ apple, grated with a pinch of ground cinnamon, or
- 1 square of melted dark chocolate drizzled over 2 tbsp smashed raspberries

Tropical fruit salad

Serves 4

Since transitioning to a vegan lifestyle fruit has fast become one of my favourite snacks in place of some of the naughtier treats I once indulged in. Tropical fruits have always been my preference, and this mixed fruit salad is a blend that includes some of my favourite varieties.

200g/7oz/1 cup mango, peeled and chopped

200g/7oz/1 cup strawberries, sliced

200g/7oz/1 cup pineapple, peeled and chopped

2 kiwis, peeled and sliced

50g/1½oz/½ cup blueberries

120ml/4fl oz/½ cup vegan coconut yoghurt

2 tbsp chia seeds

Combine all the ingredients in a bowl and devour immediately.

Quick vegan treats

- Dates
- 1 tsp nut butter eaten with a square of vegan dark chocolate or an apple
- Pre-prepared pomegranate or passionfruit seeds stirred through 2 tbsp vegan coconut yoghurt
- Vegetable crisps
- ½ avocado mashed with 1 tsp sweet chilli sauce on a cracker

How to get your kitchen vegan-ready

I'm going to tell you everything you need to keep in your cupboards to whip up delicious plant-based meals packed with flavour and nutrition.

Herbs and spices are vital because they make vegan recipes sing. Without them, and without proper seasoning, you'll be in danger of eating bland meals, which will make you more likely to crave your old diet.

My herb and spice collection has increased tenfold since I went vegan, even though I loved cooking before. Experimenting with new herbs and spices has made eating vegan feel like an exciting journey rather than a chore. A few months in, when I realized I wasn't missing meat, it contributed to a realization too. It wasn't that I'd *loved* meat in the past.

I'd loved the way it tasted when it was seasoned, marinated and prepared. I loved it in combination with the things I ate with it. I found that with a bit of culinary imagination, I was able to recreate similar flavours, and discover a whole load of new ones.

My brother, a committed meat-eater, recently came round. We were having a drink and a chat, and I prepared some plant-based nibbles: asparagus steamed with salt, pepper and a bit of garlic, and baked plantain with cumin, paprika, salt and pepper. He couldn't believe how delicious they were. Since then, he's been cooking and eating asparagus at home all the time.

10 ninja ingredients

Here are 10 essential ingredients that will turn your plant-based dishes from 'meh' to 'Mmm!'

1. Salt and black pepper: simple but essential as it brings food to life. I hated mashed potato until I tasted some that had been properly seasoned.

2. Chinese 5 spice: delicious in a stir fry, sprinkled over greens or stirred through grains with a little oil.

3. Smoked paprika: delicious in soups, stews, sprinkled over wedges, stirred into chillis. A real favourite.

4. Fresh coriander (cilantro): this aromatic herb is a favourite and gives Asian and Middle Eastern dishes a freshness I love.

5. Garam masala: the base of most of my curries, I stir this Indian spice mix through fried onions to make a base then build the curry from there.

6. Fresh rosemary: delicious roasted with baby potatoes, one of my daughter's favourites.

7. Basil: great in salads, tomato-based sauces and for home-made vegan pesto.

8. Sriracha: this spicy sauce is delicious over avocado on toast or drizzled over stir fry or my favourite peanut butter and greens stew!

9. Fresh lemon and lime juice: makes dressings sing, great in curries, and adds freshness to fruit-salad.

10. Turmeric: great with chickpea curries to give them extra flavour and that rich, vibrant colouring. Better than that, the benefits of turmeric as you now know are countless. Don't forget the black pepper.

What to keep in your store cupboard

- Quinoa
- Couscous
- Brown rice

- Wild rice
- Lentils (red, green and black)
- Egg-free noodles (buckwheat, wholewheat, rice); check all are egg-free
- Egg-free pasta
- Canned beans and pulses: black, kidney, pinto, haricot, flageolet, chickpeas
- Canned tomatoes
- Chickpea flour
- Yeast extract
- Peanut butter and nut butter

What to keep in your fridge

- Falafel
- Tofu and tempeh
- Salad leaves
- Fresh salad veg
- Veganaise
- Vegan pesto
- Caribbean hot sauce
- Sun-dried tomato paste
- Vegetable-based spread such as Vitalite

What to keep in your larder

- Onions

- Garlic

- Sweet potatoes

- Butternut squash

- Fresh chilli

- Olive oil

- Rapeseed oil (cold-pressed)

- Coconut oil

- Dried fruits and nuts

- Seed mix (hemp, flax, sesame, chia, pumpkin)

- Agave syrup

- Pine nuts

- Sriracha

- Red Thai curry paste

- Tamari

What to keep in your freezer

- Peas

- Spinach

- Leftover fresh herbs, chopped and stored in airtight containers

- Overripe bananas, cut up to use in shakes and cakes
- Emergency vegan ready-meals, such as pie or sausages, for when you get caught short
- Vegan mince of your choice (I like pea mince best)

Chapter 8

Vegan Kids

It can be hard enough getting kids to eat their fruit and veg and persuading them to broaden their repertoire beyond pizza and spaghetti bolognese. So, introducing a vegan diet into the mix may sound like an impossible challenge. Unless, of course, you're one of the lucky few who happens to have the sort of child who will eat anything (if that's you, happy days!). Otherwise, switching your children's diet to a vegan one will take some strategic planning. It's also tough to find the right way to talk to children about veganism. So many of the documentaries on the subject, for example, would be too disturbing to watch for a child. I'd give my daughter sleepless nights if I sat down and watched *Earthlings* with her. So how should you go about striking the right dietary balance, while ensuring what you serve up is going to meet with a happy reaction, and how can you find the right words to tackle the sensitive and complicated subject of ethical veganism and the health benefits of veganism without fostering disordered eating, or emotional upset?

My daughter, Myla-Grace, is seven years old. Most of the time, she lives with her mum and eats an omnivorous diet. But when she's with me, I try to feed her healthy plant-based food whenever I can. Over the past three years, since I've gone vegan, we've found some staples that she really likes, and I've tweaked the recipes of many of my favourite vegan meals to appeal to her taste.

How to talk to kids about veganism

My advice is to wait for them to ask you about it. Because they will. Myla began with the big one: 'Daddy, why are you a vegan?' That was about two years ago. Because she has a pet dog at her mum's, I explained to her that in our society, we're taught to think of some animals as pets and others as not deserving of our care. I told her that I feel we should show similar care towards pigs and cows as she does to her dog and that it doesn't make sense to me to treat some animals as 'special' while ignoring the needs of others. I told her that I believed that all animals deserved love and that because there were so many plant-based foods to choose from, I didn't feel there was any need to eat animals or animal products. Simple as that.

At the same time, I was careful not to make her feel uncomfortable or guilty about her diet. I know her maternal grandparents are sceptical about veganism, and I remember how much I loved bacon and sausages as a kid, so I try to keep a sense of perspective. On occasion, I still let her eat chicken when we eat out. But the more plant-based foods I introduce her to, the less she asks for meat.

Now Myla is older, I encourage her to get involved in the kitchen, and I've found that when she helps out with the cooking, she's far more likely to be willing to try new foods and tends to enjoy her meals more. We look through recipe books together, and I let her choose what she thinks would be tasty. In the supermarket, I let her pick up the fruit and veg and vegan products, and I'll buy what she wants, so long as it isn't too processed. I've found that introducing this element of choice and control has made her more willing to go with the vegan diet, and she's grown to take real pride in her adventurousness.

I've taken her to a city farm, and we've talked about the animals there: where different meats and dairy products come from. We used to go to the zoo and the circus, but that's all in the past. We've had several conversations about why I think they're cruel and I feel Myla is beginning to have a greater understanding. We've found alternatives, though. We visit sanctuaries at least twice a year where she can interact with animals in a way that the zoo doesn't permit. We also go on long walks with the dogs where again I talk to her about animal rights and the fact that we're all equal. I'm careful not to speak about veganism too much, and I'm aware that most of the time, Myla lives in a house where they don't share my beliefs, and that's fine.

It's been really satisfying to watch Myla's tastes evolve and see her become less picky. She now really likes some vegetables she hated before. She used to find mushrooms revolting, but now because of the way I cook them, she'll happily eat a mushroom stir fry. I also try to replicate her favourite meat-based meals when I can. I'll make vegan sausage and mash, and sometimes vegan chicken nuggets with home-made chips and salad. She's grown to enjoy salads more now and will help me pick the veg to go in her salad and chop it up.

I take Myla to Whole Foods when she's with me, and we look at the displays full of healthy food together – it makes it easier to shop with her than wandering up and down the aisles in most supermarkets where there are distracting towers of processed food everywhere. I'm well aware that for most parents, shopping in Whole Foods isn't an option, but you can get the same benefit from wandering around a traditional greengrocer or visiting the fruit and veg sellers in your local market. The bright colours, exotic varieties of fruit and colourful characters make for a fun outing, and I've found that Myla enjoys being involved in food shopping and preparation.

I think it's important not to become too rigid about veganism and remain mindful that many children have, for the most part, been conditioned to think no meal is complete without meat.

Ice cream and boiled eggs are childhood staples. Children are emotionally invested in them – they represent comfort, celebration and love. As parents, we shouldn't expect our children to miraculously switch off these associations. Forcing them to adopt a fully vegan diet overnight just because we have is likely to feel restrictive and punishing. This will be counterproductive in the long run, so it's better to take a slow and smart approach.

Five common questions

To help you along, I've answered the five most common questions parents tend to ask me when they're considering switching their family's diet.

#1 What's the key to getting kids on board with a vegan lifestyle?

Choice! Think about it. As adults, choosing to go vegan is just that: a choice. For a child with vegan parents, it might feel more like something that's been forced upon them. And nobody likes that. Also, changing our preferences, whatever our age, is a slow business. The parenting expert Noel Janis Norton says that, for most children, tasting a new food 15–20 times should be enough. However, children who are very sensitive to taste and texture may need more 'tasting sessions', and children with extreme temperaments may need to taste a food 50–100 times before they like it. Perseverance and a gradual approach is the key.

A great example is porridge. Myla refused to have plant milk with hers at first and told me it was disgusting. But gradually, I increased the ratio of oat milk to dairy, and now she doesn't have any cow's milk at all. She didn't notice the difference in taste because it changed so slowly.

#2 Are kids more at risk of deficiency from a vegan diet?

The answer to this in most cases is yes, particularly if they're already picky and aren't keen on veg. This is a valid concern, and you'll need to keep a keen eye on the nutritional balance of their meals. Supplementing with a multivitamin that contains calcium, B12 and iron is a good insurance policy, and if you're concerned that switching your child to a plant-based diet will leave them with little more than pasta with tomato sauce as a dinner option, I'd recommend introducing veganism gradually.

#3 How should you react if your child flat-out refuse to eat vegan food?

I think it's crucial to stick to your guns. Keep reminding them you're doing it because you believe in kindness to animals and keep exploring new plant-based foods with your child. Don't rise to the bait if they say things like: 'But I like eating animals!'

#4 What about eating out with kids?

The problem I often have when taking my daughter out to vegan restaurants is that it's usually a hard sell. This is down to the limited options most establishments seem to offer on the kid's menu. There's just never anything that excites her. When we're home though, she creates the menu, well at least she thinks she does. I'll always give her options, so she makes the ultimate choice, but her options are solely plant-based. On the following pages are some of her favourite dishes that go down a treat every time.

#5 How can I ensure my child gets enough nutrients?

Make sure you have a basic understanding of nutrition and what constitutes a healthy, balanced diet for your child. Know the recommended daily intake of calcium for healthy teeth and bones, and that good plant-based sources are unsweetened fortified soya milk, calcium-set tofu, cruciferous vegetables (including broccoli, cabbage and kale), pulses, whole grain bread and dried fruit (including raisins, prunes and apricots). Know what vitamins they require, including vitamin for vision, vitamin C to support the immune system, vitamin D to regulate the amount of calcium and phosphate in the body, and B12 to regulate red blood cell formation. Make sure you also educate yourself about iron and omega-3 fatty acids.

Vegan recipes kids will love

Myla's favourites are pasta, meat-free nuggets and stir fries. Check out the following recipes if you're looking for some inspiration for family meals.

Breakfast

It's morning or maybe even afternoon in my case. It's time to break the fast! Chemicals have been hard at work digesting the food in our bodies throughout our peaceful slumber. The glucose we require to power our muscles and brain is usually low first thing in the morning, and this is where a healthy nutritious breakfast steps in to replenish it. Start your day the right way.

Banana berry chia oats

Serves 1 adult and 1 child

Overnight oats have always been a favourite breakfast choice for my daughter and my niece and nephews. It's simple, convenient and packed with plenty of fruit and fibre. Since transitioning to veganism, not much has changed although I've swapped out the dairy yoghurt with vanilla plant yoghurt and they absolutely love it. Feel free to play with the fruit and discover a combination that suits you best

90g/3oz/1 cup large porridge oats

86g/3oz/½ cup chia seeds

240ml/16fl oz/1 cup plant yoghurt of choice

1 tbsp flax seeds

1 tbsp hemp seeds

1 tbsp pumpkin seeds

1 banana, chopped

2 tbsp blueberries

2 tbsp strawberries

2 tbsp raspberries

Mix the oats, chia and yoghurt together in a bowl. Sprinkle over the flax, hemp and pumpkin seeds. Leave in the refrigerator overnight.

In the morning, add the fruit and serve immediately.

Lunch

Simple, quick, tasty and packed with all the nutrients you need, these options are bound to appeal to your child's taste buds.

Smashed chickpea and avocado sandwiches

Serves 1 adult and 1 child

These sandwiches, or wraps if you prefer, make a quick lunch and often come with us on that long drive, and they always see us through.

1 × 400g/14oz can chickpeas, rinsed and drained

1 large avocado, sliced

½ small onion, finely diced

1 tbsp fresh coriander (cilantro), chopped

Juice of 1 lime

Salt and pepper to taste

Bread of choice (we usually opt for two thick slices of sourdough)

Mash the chickpeas and avocado together, Add the onion, coriander and lime juice, and mix together well. Season with salt and pepper. Spread on to bread with any chosen toppings. I sometimes add chopped tomatoes and cucumber then sprinkle a few pine nuts and pumpkin seeds.

Pesto pasta with spinach and No Chick

Serves 4 children or 1 adult and 2 children

This has to be Myla's number-one favourite dish, and you'll be pushed to find a kid who isn't a fan of pasta. She doesn't even associate it with veganism as most ingredients are things she'd ordinarily eat. This pasta dish is great served with a meat-free alternative, such as No Chick Strips. Cooked the right way you'd struggle to tell it wasn't chicken. Myla didn't have a clue. You can also use falafel instead of meat-style substitute if you prefer.

1 tbsp olive oil

3 cloves garlic, finely chopped

320g/11oz meat-style substitute (my preference is No Chick Strips)

1 vegetable stock cube

200g/7oz/2 cups pasta of your choice

½ tbsp coconut oil

3 tbsp pesto, (*see below*, or use readymade)

4 handfuls cherry tomatoes, sliced

½ tsp Italian herb seasoning

Salt and pepper to taste

1 small onion, chopped

2 carrots, peeled and chopped

1 celery stick, sliced

1 tbsp Italian seasoning

Home-made pesto

60g/2oz/3 cups fresh basil leaves

½ cup walnuts

3 tbsp vegan parmesan

juice of half a lime

3 cloves garlic, chopped

½ cup extra virgin olive oil

½ tsp cracked black pepper

½ tsp sea salt

To serve

1–2 tbsp vegan parmesan cheese, grated

Heat the olive oil in a frying pan over a medium heat. Add the chopped garlic cloves to the oil and spread evenly around the pan before throwing in the meat-substitute. Fry the meat-substitute over a medium heat for 7–8 minutes. Remove from frying pan and shred or cut into finer strips.

Bring a pot of water to boil, add the vegetable stock cube and cook the pasta according to packet directions. Strain the pasta and keep the vegetable stock to one side.

Heat the coconut oil over a medium heat, add the tomatoes and Italian seasoning, and sauté for about 5 minutes or until tender.

Prepare the pesto by adding all the ingredients to a food processor or blender and whizzing until smooth.

Place the meat-substitute and garlic in a bowl before adding the cooked pasta and tomatoes. Stir in the pesto, adding vegetable water to reach the desired consistency. Season with salt and pepper, and sprinkle over the parmesan cheese before serving.

Dinner

Who doesn't love dinner? It truly is one of life's greatest pleasures, and with the meals I have in store for you, it's going to be that much more pleasurable. There's sense of fulfilment when you take that first bite and realize that not only does it taste good but was easy to prepare too.

Sesame cauliflower with rice

Serves 1 adult and 1 child

Usually, Myla isn't one for cauliflower, well, at least not until we discovered this fantastic sesame cauliflower dish. It's packed with vitamin C, which is a powerful antioxidant, and always has her coming back for seconds. Cauliflower never tasted so good.

50g/2oz/⅓ cup plain flour

80ml/3fl oz/⅓ cup water

Salt and black pepper to taste

Pinch each of garlic and onion powder

1 small cauliflower, separated into florets

Olive oil spray

For the sauce

1 tbsp sesame oil

2 cloves garlic, finely chopped

2.5cm/½ inch fresh ginger, peeled and finely chopped

2 tbsp brown sugar/maple syrup

1 tbsp rice wine vinegar

½ tsp toasted sesame seeds

120ml/4fl oz/½ cup vegetable stock

1 tsp cornflour mixed with 1 tsp water

Preheat the oven to 180°C/350°F/gas mark 5.

Make the batter by mixing together the flour, water, garlic and onion powder, salt and pepper in a large bowl. Add the cauliflower to the bowl and gently stir until each floret is evenly coated. Use a slotted spoon to remove the cauliflower and spread evenly over a baking tray, before spraying a little oil over the cauliflower. Place in the oven and bake for 45 minutes or until golden.

To make the sauce, heat the sesame oil in a large non-stick pan over a medium heat, add the rest of the ingredients and bring to the boil before adding the cornflour and water. Reduce the heat and leave to simmer for 2–3 minutes until the sauce thickens.

Serve with your choice of rice.

Chicken-style nuggets with sweet potato fries

Serves 1 adult and 1 child

As much as I try and stay away from processed foods, I also see them as a necessity for some when transitioning. Kids love nuggets, well Myla does anyway. I first told a few fibs to get her to eat these plant-based nuggets, but now she absolutely loves them. And that's before dipping them in tomato sauce.

16 chicken-style, meat-free nuggets, cooked to packet instructions

2 large sweet potatoes, chopped

1 tbsp olive oil

2 tbsp corn starch

1 tsp garlic powder

1 tsp onion powder

1 tsp black pepper

1 tsp paprika

Slice the two sweet potatoes into evenly sized fries (not too small, not too big) You want them roughly 1cm (¼ inch) thick. Place in a large pan of cold water and soak for 30 minutes to soften and get rid of any excess starch. Rinse and drain, before patting with kitchen paper to ensure the chips are totally dry. Then add the olive oil and ensure the chips are evenly coated. Place the fries on a baking tray lined with parchment paper to avoid fries sticking to the pan.

Whisk together the corn starch, garlic powder, onion powder, black pepper and paprika. Sprinkle the dry mix over the fries. Holding off on the salt till the end will assist in your fries, staying super crispy.

Bake in a preheated oven 220°C/425°F/gas mark 7 for 20 minutes or until crispy, flipping the fries halfway through cooking. When cooked, add salt to taste if required.

These fries are great served with meat-free, chicken-style nuggets. I also make a little side salad with her favourite fruits and vegetables.

Chapter 9

Help! What If...

By going vegan, you're making a significant change to your lifestyle. There may be times that it feels like a bumpy road, and as with any shifts in habit, there may be obstacles and distractions that throw you off course. This chapter is here to help you plan, with advice on what you can do to ensure you stay on track. The 'what ifs' here are based on situations I've experienced myself, and on dilemmas my clients have shared with me. You may recognize some of them from your own experience, too.

What if I'm caught out on the road, or at work, with no vegan options?

Preparation is the key to success. This is true whether you're planning a presentation, getting ready for a job interview, or running a marathon. It's equally valid of changing your diet. Finding yourself out and about, ill-prepared, with temptation all around is enough to test even the most committed vegan. I must report that in the years since I went plant-based, the vegan food scene has exploded, and also the most mainstream chain cafés and restaurants now offer options. So, the good news is that if you do find yourself caught out, at least there will be more than a side salad and portion of chips to choose from. Even if there isn't something strictly vegan on the menu, most tasty veggie options can be made vegan (or veganized) with a few tweaks.

Chain cafés that offer vegan options include:

- Pizza Express
- Zizzi
- Franco Manca
- Bill's
- Giraffe
- Wagamama

And if you're really at a loose end and desperate times call for desperate measures:

- Subway
- Burger King
- McDonald's

What if a dinner-party host puts a plate of chicken in front of me?

Well, I certainly wouldn't eat it! If I know I'm going to a dinner party, I always plan and usually try to inform the host about my diet. If the host seems concerned and 'put out', which does sometimes happen, I always suggest bringing my own vegan alternative to be served up with everyone else's meal. In the worst-case scenario, I leave the chicken or offer it to another guest and enjoy double servings of veg. There's no need to make a fuss, just be polite and keep smiling.

Great, quick things to take along to a dinner party:

- Falafel
- A pre-prepared nut roast or vegan pie that just needs reheating
- A vegan ready meal (you'll find lots of delicious plant-based options in the fresh and frozen cabinets of your local supermarket)
- Vegan sausages

What if I get pregnant?

That's great news!! And you can continue with your vegan diet and have a happy, healthy pregnancy and an even happier healthy baby. Vegan mums-to-be need to ensure they get enough iron, B12, calcium and vitamin D, so make sure you include lots of pulses in your diet, along with plenty of dark green leafy veg. Speak to your doctor or midwife about the best B12 and vitamin D supplements to take during your pregnancy.

Bump-friendly vegan foods to fill up on:

- Pulses
- Asparagus

- Beetroot
- Leafy greens
- Marmite or Vegemite
- Fortified unsweetened soya milk
- Sesame seeds and tahini
- Broccoli

What if my doctor says I'm anaemic – is it due to my vegan diet?

There is no getting away from the fact that choosing a vegan diet and not eating correctly can lead to an iron deficiency, but you don't need to abandon your lifestyle choice to get your iron levels up. A little more attention to the nutritional balance of your diet should restore your levels. Supplement with a multivitamin that contains iron and B12, which you can't get from vegan food sources, and you'll be covering all the bases. Try upping your intake of the following iron-rich vegan foods:

- Dried fruit
- Brown rice
- Nuts and seeds
- Lentils and beans
- Tofu and tempeh
- Edamame beans

What if I can't find vegan-friendly clothing?

This can be tricky and at times, frustrating. When I first began my journey, I struggled to find footwear and was usually left with cheap shoes that rubbed my feet raw. I also had to find alternatives to my leather jackets and belts, the struggle was real! Most shops would have lots of vegan options, but these were inferior quality (not my style) or ridiculously expensive and unappealing, to say the least. The only way I eventually overcame was by researching and, in doing so, I found some great 100 per cent ethical and vegan clothing companies. So, get on Google and make it a fun part of your journey.

This is a list of inspiring brands and ranges offering vegan, sustainable and ethical products worth checking out:

- Beyond Skin (high-end shoes): www.beyond-skin.com
- Matt & Nat (bags and wallets): https://mattandnat.com
- Veja (vegan clothing range): www.veja-store.com
- Toms (vegan clothing range): www.toms.com
- Dr Martens (vegan range of boots and shoes): www.drmartens.com
- Saucony (vegan clothing range): www.saucony.com
- Mamoq (fashions, jewellery and accessories): www.mamoq.com
- We Are Thought (vegan clothing range): www.wearethought.com

What if there's no vegan option on a long-haul flight?

I've suffered from severe hunger and settled for bread rolls on certain flights due to not being prepared. Although the vegan movement is becoming more and more widespread all the time, some organizations simply haven't caught up. The answer to this is to prepare your own flight-friendly food. Things that are easy to eat, don't require heating and aren't too bulky. I always take on board spinach, falafel and avocado wraps or stuffed pittas!

Some airlines will provide a vegan meal if you ask in advance. Their online booking systems will let you specify; for others, you'll need to call customer services after you've booked your ticket and flag your request again at check-in.

The following airlines should provide an excellent vegan meal[1]:

- Asiana
- Dragonair
- Bangkok Airways
- Singapore Airlines
- South African Airways
- Air China
- Air India
- Cathay Pacific
- Korean Air

- Iberia

- Qatar Airways

- Turkish Airlines

- British Airways

- Air France

- United Airlines

- American Airlines

- KLM

What if I'm overseas and there are no vegan options?

I recommend you always do your research before flying abroad. I'd also learn how to say, and even explain, that you're vegan in the language of the country you're visiting: *vegano: niente carne, niente pesce, niente uova, niente latte, niente formaggio*. That's Italian for 'vegan: no meat, no fish, no eggs, no dairy, no cheese'. I'm in Brindisi, Italy, as I'm writing this, and I arrived well aware that vegan options in this area would be limited, so I came prepared. With the Internet at your fingertips, it's so easy to discover vegan options in many places, although I grant you, not everywhere. Keep a note of vegan-friendly cafés and restaurants, book tables for evening meals and if you're going to stay with somebody, let your hosts know that you're eating vegan. Whenever I've travelled to countries that haven't been vegan-friendly, I've simply planned grocery visits to stores according to the meals I want to prepare, as I do at home. The Vegan Society website (www.vegansociety.com/lifestyle/travel) is an excellent place to start your research.

What if people lecture me about why I need meat?

The stereotype that we vegans face can be daunting at times. Family and friends may well worry about our health, as there is widespread misinformation and ignorance about vegan eating. Culturally, vegans are often perceived as weak, forever hungry and nutrient deficient, and when we say we're vegan, the 'eye-rolls' may grate.

If you have the misfortune of being surrounded by colleagues, friends or family who seem to want to lecture you endlessly about the potential dangers of avoiding meat and dairy, it can be irritating and exhausting. But I've often found that behind the knee-jerk dismissal is a genuine curiosity and willingness to find out more about vegan eating. Depending on who I'm talking to, I try to find out whether they want to have a discussion, or just talk at me. I either nod my head and smile or engage in a healthy debate in which we share our different points of view. If you're going for the second option, it's essential to do your research about veganism so you can give clear facts. It's always good to bring it back to the person too.

I've found the best approach is simply to ignore the negativity and stay positive and inspiring. Show your friends and family how amazing you feel. Cook for them whenever you can so they can see your food choices are vibrant, tasty and fun. Last, never judge or get defensive; it doesn't work and can lead to people being more judgemental and negative. If they refuse to leave it alone, try one of the following conversation finishers:

- 'Each to their own, anyway, let's talk about something else!'

- 'I'd love to talk more about this another time, but I'm more interested in finding out about what's going on with you.'

- 'It's a diet that works for me, anyway. I'm sure yours works for you too.'

When things get heated, bring it back to the personal. It's harder for somebody to lecture you when you explain you've made a deeply personal choice (and the subtext is: 'This really has nothing to do with you or your opinions.'). End of.

What if I *really* crave a non-vegan food?

You're human, so it's going to happen. Having said that, it's less likely to be a problem if you don't allow yourself to get too hungry. Whenever I'm tempted to give in to the urge to eat something that contains animal products, I always revert to reminding myself of why I made the transition. Chocolate is my biggest temptation. I was previously a chocoholic. Lindt, Cadbury Dairy Milk and Buttons, Bounty bars, you name it, I was eating it. So, at first, I did suffer some severe cravings. When they got intense, I'd make myself watch a bit of the *Earthlings* documentary to remember why I'd decided to go vegan. If you remind yourself of your motivation for change, your 'why', then your willpower will be stronger than any passing desire you might feel for chocolate, a cheesy pizza or a roast dinner.

What if I eat non-vegan food?

Digest it, get rid of it, and now you know for next time. Whether it's by mistake or a temporary slip in willpower, mistakes will be made. You've taken a big step in changing your lifestyle for the greater good. Don't give yourself a hard time or feel like you've let yourself down. Next time, you'll be more aware. Focus on all the positive changes you've made, and don't sweat the small slip-ups if you make them.

Conclusion

The human body is one of the most complex machines on this planet, yet we abuse our bodies every day in the name of taste, habit, culture and convenience. I've eaten my fair share of junk food over the years and, admittedly, I still have the occasional treat. But here's the thing: it's not a treat! In fact it's just the opposite.

There is much resistance to change in our world, but I believe that more and more of us will wake up and see what we're doing, not only to ourselves but to innocent animals and our planet. This journey begins with love and compassion for yourself. Respect your amazing machine – it's the only one you have – and don't wait to get sick before you contemplate a lifestyle change.

Could you eat a plant-based diet one day a week? If the answer is 'yes', then start there. Start wherever you can. The most important thing is that you start. Now is the perfect time to affect change in your life, to begin a journey of love, compassion, consciousness, health and growth. I know the thought of changing habits of a lifetime can seem daunting, but the results will be so worth it. Let's do this!

Following my Fit Vegan plan will restore balance in your life. Prepare to train, eat and adopt a lifestyle based on achieving total fitness, health and wellbeing; a fitter, faster, stronger you! Once you've made a conscious choice to give your body the nutrition it needs to perform at an optimum level and remain in good health, the beautiful journey begins. Let me guide you as you take these positive steps towards total fitness.

I'm so excited for you, and after just a few weeks of following my plan you'll begin to understand why: as you reap the benefits of a plant based diet you'll become a better version of yourself. You'll be choosing a lifestyle that causes the least harm possible – to your health, to the environment and to innocent animals. That choice will be greatly rewarded.

Too often I have witnessed close friends and family members willing to make a change when it was too late. Please don't be that person. I chose vegan because I love and value all living beings. Vegan because it felt like the right thing to do. Vegan because I have never felt better within myself. Vegan for animals. Vegan for my health. Vegan for our planet, and vegan for the rest of my life. Veganism has enriched my life and I simply want the same for you. Begin this journey with your *why* and watch it fuel your fire for change as you become the Fit Vegan.

Appendix

The Fit Vegan Workout Plan

After each set, continue on to the next. When you can complete 10 sets without resting, it's time to scale up to the next level.

	Phase A: Weeks 1–4		
	Week 1		
	Advanced	**Intermediate**	**Beginner**
Workout 1 × 10 sets	5 pull-ups 10 press-ups 15 air squats	5 ring rows 10 incline press-ups 15 air squats	3 ring rows 7 incline press-ups 10 air squats
Workout 2 × 4 sets	30-second handstand 30-second dead hang 30-second half plank 30m bear crawl	30-second front support hold 30-second dead hang supported 30-second half plank 30m bear crawl	30-second front support hold 30-second ring row supported 30-second half plank knees down 30-second plank
Workout 3 × 3 sets	400m run 15 broad jumps 15 kettlebell swings	Scale run length to 200m and weight of kettlebell swing	
Workout 4	50 burpees for time	30 burpees	20 burpees (scale if needed)

	Week 2		
	Advanced	**Intermediate**	**Beginner**
Workout 1	For time: 50 pull-ups 50 press-ups 50 sit-ups 50 air squats	Scale pull-ups to ring rows Scale press-ups to incline press-ups Reduce reps for sit-ups and air squats	
Workout 2	50 DUBs[1]/50 sit-ups 40 DUBs/40 sit-ups 30 DUBs/30 sit-ups 20 DUBs/20 sit-ups 10 DUBs/10 sit-ups	100 singles[2] 50 sit-ups 80 singles 40 sit-ups 60 singles 30 sit-ups 40 singles 20 sit-ups 10 DUBS or 20 singles 10 sit-ups	75 singles 30 sit-ups 60 singles 20 sit-ups 60 singles 15 sit-ups 40 singles 10 sit-ups 10 DUBs or 20 singles 10 sit-ups
Workout 3	× 10 reps 100m sprint or high knees running in place 10 burpees	× 7 reps 100m sprint 10 burpees	× 5 reps 100m sprint 8 burpees
Workout 4 **× 3 sets**	20 alternate lunges 20 kettlebell swings 40m single-arm farmer's carry	Scale the weight and lunges with support if needed	

[1] DUBs (Double Unders): exercise with a skipping rope in which the participant jumps higher than normal while swinging the rope twice under their feet, i.e. double under.

[2] Singles: as for Double Unders, but the rope passes just once under the participant's feet.

	Week 3		
	Advanced	**Intermediate**	**Beginner**
Workout 1 × 3 sets	400m run 50 sit-ups 50m bear crawl	200m run 30 sit-ups 30m bear crawl	100m run 20 sit-ups 20m bear crawl
Workout 2	12-9-3 dumbbell or kettlebell thrusters/ burpees	Adjust weights and scale burpees if needed	
Workout 3 × 5 sets	10 pull-ups 15 press-ups 20 sit-ups 25 air squats	Scale pull-ups to ring rows Scale press-ups to incline press-ups Reduce reps for sit-ups and air squats	
Workout 4 × 3 sets	30-second handstand hold 30-second single-arm kettlebell hold (each side) 30-second V-sit	30-second front support hold 30-second single-arm kettlebell hold (each side) 30-second floor V-sit, hands by knees	30-second front support hold 30-second single-arm kettlebell hold (each side) 30-second floor V-sit, hands by thighs
	Week 4		
	Advanced	**Intermediate**	**Beginner**
Workout 1 × 4 sets	200m run 30 air squats	200m run 20 air squats	100m run 20 air squats
Workout 2 × 10 sets	6 burpees 6 pull-ups	6 burpees 6 ring rows	
Workout 3 × 3 sets	50m bear crawl 20 kettlebell deadlifts (heavy double kettlebell deadlifts) 10 broad jumps	30m bear crawl 10 kettlebell deadlifts (heavy double kettlebell deadlifts) 5 broad jumps	Scale weight and length of bear crawl
Workout 4 × 3 sets	60-second dead hang 60-second at the bottom of kettlebell front squat 60-second standing kettlebell hold	Scale weight to suit Scale dead hang to standing kettlebell by side hold or supported dead hang	

	Phase B Week 5-8		
	Week 5		
	Advanced	**Intermediate**	**Beginner**
Workout 1 **× 15 sets**	5 pull-ups 5 dips 10 press-ups 15 air squats	5 ring rows 5 dips 10 incline press-ups 15 air squats	3 ring rows 3 dips 7 incline press-ups 10 air squats
Workout 2 **× 4 sets**	45-second handstand 45-second dead hang 30-second half plank 30m bear crawl	45-second front support hold 45-second dead hang supported 45-second half plank 45m bear crawl	45-second front support hold 45-second ring row supported 45-second half plank knee down 45-second plank
Workout 3 **× 3 sets**	600m run 20 broad jump 20 kettlebell swings	Scale run length to 400m and weight of kettlebell swings	
Workout 4	75 burpees for time	50 burpees	30 burpees

	Week 6		
	Advanced	**Intermediate**	**Beginner**
Workout 1	75 pull-ups 75 press-ups 75 sit-ups 75 air squats	Scale pull-ups to ring rows Scale press-ups to incline press-ups Reduce reps for sit-ups and air squats	
Workout 2	50 DUBs/50 sit-ups 40 DUBs/40 sit-ups 30 DUBs/30 sit-ups 20 DUBs/20 sit-ups 10 DUBs/10 sit-ups	100 singles 50 sit-ups 80 singles 40 sit-ups 60 singles 30 sit-ups 40 singles 20 sit-ups 10 DUBs or 20 singles 10 sit-ups	75 singles 30 sit-ups 60 singles 20 sit-ups 60 singles 15 sit-ups 40 singles 10 sit-ups 10 DUBs or 20 singles 10 sit-ups
Workout 3 × 10 sets	100m sprint 10 burpees	100m sprint 10 burpees	100m sprint 8 burpees
Workout 4 × 3 sets	20 step-ups 30 kettlebell swings 60m single-arm farmer's carry	Scale the weight and lunges with support if needed	

	Week 7		
	Advanced	**Intermediate**	**Beginner**
Workout 1 × 3 sets	600m run 75 sit-ups 75m bear crawl	400m run 50 sit-ups 50m bear crawl	200m run 30 sit-ups 30m bear crawl
Workout 2	15-12-6[3] kettlebell/ dumbbell thrusters and burpees	Adjust weights and scale burpees if needed	
Workout 3 × 5 sets	15 pull-ups 20 press-ups 25 sit-ups 30 air squats	Scale pull-ups to ring rows Scale press-ups to incline press-ups Reduce reps for sit-ups and air squats	
Workout 4 × 4 sets	30-second handstand hold 30-second single-arm kettlebell hold (each side) 30-second V-sit	30-second front support hold 30-second single-arm kettlebell hold (each side) 30-second floor V-sit, hands by knees	30-second front support hold 30-second single-arm kettlebell hold (each side) 30-second floor V-sit, hands by thighs

[3] 15 kettlebell/dumbbell thrusters and burpees, followed by 12, followed by 6

	Week 8		
	Advanced	**Intermediate**	**Beginner**
Workout 1 **× 4 sets**	300m run 30 air squats	200m run 30 air squats	200m run 20 air squats
Workout 2 **× 10 sets**	8 burpees 8 pull-ups	8 burpees 8 ring rows	
Workout 3	× 4 reps 50m bear crawl 20 kettlebell deadlifts (heavy double kettlebell deadlifts) 10 broad jumps	× 3 reps 50m bear crawl 20 kettlebell deadlifts (heavy double kettlebell deadlifts) 10 broad jumps	Scale weight and length of bear crawl
Workout 4 **× 3 sets**	90-second dead hang 90-second at the bottom of kettlebell front squat 90-second standing kettlebell hold	Scale weight to suit Scale dead hang to standing kettlebell by side hold or supported dead hang	

Phase C: Weeks 9-12			
Week 9			
	Advanced	**Intermediate**	**Beginner**
Workout 1	AMRAP[4] 20 5 pull-ups 10 press-ups 15 air squats	AMRAP 20 5 ring rows 10 incline press-ups 15 air squats	AMRAP 15 5 ring rows 10 incline press-ups 15 air squats
Workout 2 × 4 sets	60-second handstand 60-second dead hang 60-second half plank 60m bear crawl	60-second in front support hold 60-second dead hang supported 60-second half plank 60m bear crawl	60-second in front support hold 60-second ring row supported 60-second half plank 60-second plank
Workout 3 × 3 sets	800m run 30 broad jumps 30 kettlebell swings	Scale run length to 600m and weight of kettlebell swing	
Workout 4	For time: 100 burpees	For time: 75 burpees	For time: 50 burpees

[4] AMRAP: as many reps as possible. Usually followed by a number to indicate the time period in which to complete the reps, e.g. AMRAP 15 = as many reps as possible in 15 minutes.

	Week 10		
	Advanced	**Intermediate**	**Beginner**
Workout 1	For time: 100 pull-ups 100 press-ups 100 sit-ups 100 air squats	Scale pull-ups to ring rows Scale press-ups to incline press-ups Reduce reps for sit-ups and air squats	
Workout 2	50 DUBs/50 sit-ups 40 DUBs/40 sit-ups 30 DUBs/30 sit-ups 20 DUBs/20 sit-ups 10 DUBs/10 sit-ups	100 singles 50 sit-ups 80 singles 40 sit-ups 60 singles 30 sit-ups 40 singles 20 sit-ups 10 DUBs or 20 singles 10 sit-ups	75 singles 30 sit-ups 60 singles 20 sit-ups 60 singles 15 sit-ups 40 singles 10 sit-ups 10 DUBs or 20 singles 10 sit-ups
Workout 3 × 10 sets	100m sprint 12 burpees	100m sprint 10 burpees	100m sprint 8 burpees
Workout 4 × 3 sets	20 weighted step-ups 30 kettlebell swings 80m single-arm farmer's carry	Scale the weight and lunges with support if needed	

	Week 11		
	Advanced	**Intermediate**	**Beginner**
Workout 1 × 3 sets	800m run 100 sit-ups 100m bear crawl	600m run 75 sit-ups 75m bear crawl	400m run 50 sit-ups 50m bear crawl
Workout 2	21-15-9 dumbbell or kettlebell thrusters/ burpees	Adjust weights and scale burpees if needed	
Workout 3 × 5 sets	20 pull-ups 30 press-ups 40 sit-ups 50 air squats	Scale pull-ups to ring rows Scale press-ups to incline press-ups Reduce reps for sit-ups and air squats	
Workout 4 x5 sets	30-second handstand hold 30-second single-arm kettlebell hold (each side) 30-second V-sit	30-second front support hold 30-second single-arm kettlebell hold (each side) 30-second floor V-sit, hands by knees	30-second front support hold 30-second single-arm kettlebell hold (each side) 30-second floor V-sit, hands by thighs
	Week 12		
	Advanced	**Intermediate**	**Beginner**
Workout 1 × 4 sets	400m run 40 squats	300m run 30 squats	200m run 30 squats
Workout 2 × 10 sets	10 burpees 10 pull-ups	10 burpees 10 ring rows	
Workout 3	× 5 reps 50m bear crawl 20 kettlebell deadlifts (heavy double kettlebell deadlifts) 10 broad jumps	× 4 reps 50m bear crawl 20 kettlebell deadlifts (heavy double kettlebell deadlifts) 10 broad jumps	Scale weight and length of bear crawl
Workout 4 × 3 sets	120-second dead hang 120-second bottom of kettlebell front squat 120-second standing kettlebell hold	Scale weight to suit Scale dead hang to standing kettlebell by side hold or supported dead hang	

References

Chapter 1: More Than Just Fruit and Veg

1. Elsevier (2019), 'More than a diet': www.thelancet.com/journals/lanplh/article/PIIS2542-5196(19)30023-3/fulltext [Accessed 15 August 2019]

2. University of Oxford (2016), 'Veggie-based diets could save 8 million lives by 2050 and cut global warming': www.ox.ac.uk/news/2016-03-22-veggie-based-diets-could-save-8-million-lives-2050-and-cut-global-warming [Accessed 15 August 2019]

3. GlobalData (2018), 'How UK consumers identify their dietary requirements and what drives their decision': http://client.globaldata.com/static/PR3371.png [Accessed 15 August 2019]

4. GlobalData (2018), 'Almost half of vegans made the switch within the last year': www.retail-insight-network.com/comment/vegan-switch-numbers/ [Accessed 15 August 2019]

5. Hormes, J. and Heill, S. (2018), 'Is There A Link Between Your Pets and Your Food Choices?': www.albany.edu/news/86282.php [Accessed 15 August 2019]

Chapter 2: No-Meat Muscle

1. *The Economist* (2018), 'Why people in rich countries are eating more vegan food': www.economist.com/briefing/2018/10/13why-people-in-rich-countries-are-eating-more-vegan-food [Accessed 15 August 2019]

2. Harvard Health Publishing (2018), 'When it comes to protein, how much is too much?': www.health.harvard.edu/diet-and-weight-loss/when-it-comes-to-protein-how-much-is-too-much [Accessed 15 August 2019]

3. Wilson, B. (2019), 'Protein mania: the rich world's new diet obsession': www.theguardian.com/news/2019/jan/04/protein-mania-the-rich-worlds-new-diet-obsession [Accessed 15 August 2019]

4. Morton, R.W., et al. (2018), 'A systematic review, meta-analysis and meta-regression of the effect of protein supplementation on resistance training-induced gains in muscle mass and strength in healthy adults': www.ncbi.nlm.nih.gov/pubmed/28698222 [Accessed 15 August 2019]

5. Craig, W.J. (1994), 'Iron status of vegetarians': www.ncbi.nlm.nih.gov/pubmed/8172127 [Accessed 15 August 2019]

6. Ibid.

7. Craig, W.J. (1994), 'Health effects of vegan diets', *The American Journal of Clinical Nutrition*, Volume 89, Issue 5, May 2009, pages 1627S–1633S

8. Lang, S. (2005), 'Lactose intolerance seems linked to ancestral struggles with harsh climate and cattle diseases': http://news.cornell.edu/stories/2005/06/lactose-intolerance-linked-ancestral-struggles-climate-diseases [Accessed 15 August 2019]

9. Winham, D.M. and Hutchins, A.M. (2011), 'Perceptions of flatulence from bean consumption among adults in 3 feeding studies': www.ncbi.nlm.nih.gov/pmc/articles/PMC3228670/ [Accessed 15 August 2019]

10. Domínguez, R. et al. (2017), 'Effects of Beetroot Juice Supplementation on Cardiorespiratory Endurance in Athletes. A Systematic Review': www.ncbi.nlm.nih.gov/pmc/articles/PMC5295087/ [Accessed 15 August 2019]

11. University of Exeter (2009), 'Beetroot Juice Boosts Stamina, New Study Shows': www.sciencedaily.com/releases/2009/08/090806141520.htm [Accessed 15 August 2019]

12. Hoffman, J.R. and Falvo, M.J. (2004), 'Protein – Which is Best?': www.ncbi.nlm.nih.gov/pmc/articles/PMC3905294/ [Accessed 15 August 2019]

13. Singh, P. et al. (2008), 'Functional and Edible Uses of Soy Protein Products': https://onlinelibrary.wiley.com/doi/full/10.1111/j.1541-4337.2007.00025.x [Accessed 15 August 2019]

14. Pollan, M. (2009), *In Defense of Food: An Eater's Manifesto*. Penguin Books.

15. Benedict, F.G. and Roth, P. (1915), 'The metabolism of vegetarians as compared with the metabolism of non-vegetarians of like weight and height': www.jbc.org/content/20/3/231.full.pdf [Accessed 15 August 2019]

16. Greger, M. (2018), 'The First Studies on Vegetarian Athletes': https://nutritionfacts.org/video/the-first-studies-on-vegetarian-athletes/ [Accessed 15 August 2019]

17. *The New York Times* (1907), 'Vegetarians the Stronger: Yale's Flesh-Eating Athletes Beaten in Severe Endurance Tests': www.nytimes.com/1907/03/22/archives/vegetarians-the-stronger-yales-flesheating-athletes-beaten-in.html [Accessed 15 August 2019]

Chapter 3: Healthy Choices

1. Wighton, K. (2017), 'Eating more fruits and vegetables may prevent millions of premature deaths': www.imperial.ac.uk/news/177778/eating-more-fruits-vegetables-prevent-millions/ [Accessed 15 August 2019]

2. Oyebode, O. (2014), 'UCL study finds new evidence linking fruit and vegetable consumption with lower mortality': www.ucl.ac.uk/news/2014/apr/ucl-study-finds-new-evidence-linking-fruit-and-vegetable-consumption-lower-mortality [Accessed 15 August 2019] Full Fact (2018), 'How much meat do we eat?': https://fullfact.org/health/vegetarian-vegan-uk/ [Accessed 15 August 2019]

3. Viva! Health (2019), 'Don't Feed Cancer': www.vivahealth.org.uk/veganhealth/dont-feed-cancer [Accessed 15 August 2019]

4. Prostate.net (2019), 'Can A Plant Based Diet Reverse Prostate Cancer?': https://prostate.net/articles/plant-based-diet-may-reverse-prostate-cancer/ [Accessed 15 August 2019]

5. Esselstyn, C.B. (2017), 'A plant-based diet and coronary artery disease: a mandate for effective therapy': https://www.ncbi.nlm.nih.gov/pmc/articles/PMC5466936/ [Accessed 15 August 2019]

6. Craig, W.J. and Mangels, A.R. (2009), 'Position of the American Dietetic Association: Vegetarian Diets, *Journal of the American Dietetic Association*, 1985; 109(7); 1266–82

7. Boseley, S. (2015), 'Processed meats rank alongside smoking as cancer causes – WHO': www.theguardian.com/society/2015/

oct/26/bacon-ham-sausages-processed-meats-cancer-risk-
smoking-says-who?CMP=share_btn_link [Accessed 15 August
2019]

8. NHS (2018), 'Processed meats like bacon may increase breast
   cancer risk': www.nhs.uk/news/cancer/processed-meats-bacon-
   may-increase-breast-cancer-risk/ [Accessed 15 August 2019]

9. Wilson, B. (2018), 'Yes, bacon really is killing us': www.
   theguardian.com/news/2018/mar/01/bacon-cancer-processed-
   meats-nitrates-nitrites-sausages [Accessed 15 August 2019]

10. Harvard Health Publishing, 'What's the beef with red meat?':
    www.health.harvard.edu/healthbeat/whats-the-beef-with-red-
    meat [Accessed 15 August 2019]

11. Etemadi, A. (2017), 'Mortality from different causes associated
    with meat, heme iron, nitrates, and nitrites in the NIH-AARP Diet
    and Health Study: population based cohort study': www.bmj.
    com/content/357/bmj.j1957 [Accessed 15 August 2019]

12. Greger, M. How Not to Die: Discover the Foods Scientifically
    Proven to Prevent and Reverse Disease (Pan Macmillan, 2016):
    187

13. Lawrence, F. (2013), 'Supermarkets selling chicken that is nearly
    a fifth water': www.theguardian.com/world/2013/dec/06/
    supermarket-frozen-chicken-breasts-water [Accessed 15 August
    2019]

14. Wang, Y. et al. (2010), 'Modern organic and broiler chickens
    sold for human consumption provide more energy from fat than
    protein', Public Health Nutrition, 2010; 13(3), 400–8

15. Rivera, L. 2017), 'Unmasking the truth behind food labelling in
    the chicken industry': www.independent.co.uk/life-style/food-
    and-drink/supermarket-chicken-labels-truth-free-range-battery-
    treatment-organic-a7751536.html [Accessed 15 August 2019]

16. Greger, M. How Not to Die: Discover the Foods Scientifically
    Proven to Prevent and Reverse Disease (Pan Macmillan, 2016):
    187

17. Aune, D. et al. (2009), 'Egg consumption and the risk of cancer: a
    multisite case-control study in Uruguay': www.ncbi.nlm.nih.gov/
    pubmed/20104980 [Accessed 15 August 2019]

18. Abdelhamid, A.S. et al. (2018), 'Omega-3 fatty acids for the
    primary and secondary prevention of cardiovascular disease',

http://cochranelibrary-wiley.com/doi/10.1002/14651858.
CD003177.pub3/full [Accessed 15 August 2019]

19. Robinson Simon, D., '5 Reasons You Should Stop Eating Salmon':
www.mindbodygreen.com/0-14180/5-reasons-you-should-stop-
eating-salmon.html [Accessed 15 August 2019]

20. Smith, M. et al. (2018), 'Microplastics in Seafood and the
Implications for Human Health': www.ncbi.nlm.nih.gov/pmc/
articles/PMC6132564/ [Accessed 15 August 2019]

21. Michaëlsson, K. et al. (2014), 'Milk intake and risk of mortality
and fractures in women and men: cohort studies': www.bmj.com/
content/349/bmj.g6015 [Accessed 15 August 2019]

Chapter 4: Do Good, Feel Good

1. Bosely, S. (2017), '"Pro-vegetarian" diet could halve chance
of obesity': www.theguardian.com/society/2017/may/19/pro-
vegetarian-diet-halve-chance-obesity?CMP=soc_567 [Accessed
15 August 2019]

2. University of Oxford (2018), 'New estimates of the environmental
cost of food': www.ox.ac.uk/news/2018-06-01-new-estimates-
environmental-cost-food [Accessed 15 August 2019]

3. Madigan, M. and Karhu, E. (2018), 'The role of plant-based
nutrition in cancer prevention': https://jumdjournal.net/article/
view/2892 [Accessed 15 August 2019]

4. Paddock, C. (2009), 'Vegetarians Have Lower Cancer Risk,
UK Study': www.medicalnewstoday.com/articles/155965.php
[Accessed 15 August 2019]

5. Kay, T.J. et al. (2009), 'Cancer incidence in British vegetarians':
www.nature.com/articles/6605098 [Accessed 15 August 2019]

6. Juhl, C.R. et al. (2018), 'Dairy Intake and Acne Vulgaris: A
Systematic Review and Meta-Analysis of 78,529 Children,
Adolescents, and Young Adults': www.ncbi.nlm.nih.gov/pmc/
articles/PMC6115795/ [Accessed 15 August 2019]

7. Beezhold, B. (2018), 'Vegans report less stress and anxiety than
omnivores': www.ncbi.nlm.nih.gov/pubmed/25415255 [Accessed
15 August 2019]

8. Scarborough, P. et al. (2014), 'Dietary greenhouse gas emissions
of meat-eaters, fish-eaters, vegetarians and vegans in the UK':

https://link.springer.com/article/10.1007%2Fs10584-014-1169-1 [Accessed 15 August 2019]

9. Friedman, L. et al. (2018), 'The Meat Question, by the Numbers': www.nytimes.com/2018/01/25/climate/cows-global-warming.html [Accessed 15 August 2019]

10. Pleasance, C. (2015), 'We really are a nation of meat eaters: Carnivores devour more than 7,000 animals in their lifetime including 11 cows, 2,400 chickens and 30 sheep': www.dailymail.co.uk/news/article-2985910/We-really-nation-meat-eaters-Carnivores-devour-7-000-animals-life-time-including-11-cows-2-400-chickens-30-sheep.html [Accessed 15 August 2019]

11. Ricard, M. (2013), 'On Keeping a Vegan or Vegetarian Diet': www.youtube.com/watch?v=n7T7vZr0c6s [Accessed 15 August 2019]

12. University of Oxford (2018), 'New estimates of the environmental cost of food': www.ox.ac.uk/news/2018-06-01-new-estimates-environmental-cost-food [Accessed 15 August 2019]

13. Carrington, D. (2018), 'Avoiding meat and dairy is "single biggest way" to reduce your impact on Earth': www.theguardian.com/environment/2018/may/31/avoiding-meat-and-dairy-is-single-biggest-way-to-reduce-your-impact-on-earth [Accessed 15 August 2019]

14. Pittman, A. (2017), 'How Planting Crops Used to Feed Livestock is Contributing to Habitat Destruction': www.onegreenplanet.org/environment/livestock-feed-and-habitat-destruction [Accessed 15 August 2019]

15. Bar-On, Y.M. (2018), 'The biomass distribution on Earth': www.pnas.org/content/115/25/6506 [Accessed 15 August 2019]

16. Food and Agriculture Organization of the United Nations (2013), 'Major cuts of greenhouse gas emissions from livestock within reach' www.fao.org/news/story/en/item/197623/icode/ [Accessed 15 August 2019]

17. University of Twente (2011), 'Calculating water footprints of animal, plant proteins': https://phys.org/news/2011-01-footprints-animal-proteins.html [Accessed 15 August 2019]

18. Wilson, L. (2013), 'The carbon foodprint of 5 diets compared': http://shrinkthatfootprint.com/food-carbon-footprint-diet [Accessed 15 August 2019]

19. Veganuary.com: Chickens and Hens: Reasons to Try Vegan':
    https://veganuary.com/why/animals/chickens/ [Accessed
    15 August 2019]
20. Forks Over Knives.com, 'Forks Over Knives: The Documentary
    Feature': www.forksoverknives.com/the-film/#gs.qcwgt1 [Accessed
    15 August 2019]
21. Cowspiracy.com, 'Cowspiracy: The Sustainability Secret': www.
    cowspiracy.com/facts [Accessed 15 August 2019]

Chapter 5: Where to Start

1. Rowlat, J. (2007), 'Does your daily bread contain human hair?':
   www.bbc.co.uk/blogs/newsnight/2007/01/does_your_daily_
   bread_contain_human_hair.html [Accessed 15 August 2019]

Chapter 9: Help! What If...

1. Hines, N (2019), 'The best and worst airlines for vegetarians and
   vegans': https://matadornetwork.com/read/best-worst-airlines-
   vegetarians-vegans/ [Accessed 15 August 2019]

Resources

Documentaries

Cowspiracy (2014)

Dominion (2018)

Earthlings (2005)

The End of Meat (2017)

Food Choices (2016)

Food Matters (2008)

Forks Over Knives (2011)

The Game Changers (2019)

Got the Facts on Milk? (2011)

Land of Hope and Glory (2017)

Live and Let Live (2013)

Vegucated (2011)

What the Health (2017)

Books

The China Study: The Most Comprehensive Study of Nutrition Ever Conducted and the Startling Implications for Diet, Weight Loss, and Long-term Health, T. Colin Campbell (BenBella Books, 2006)

How Not to Die: Discover the Foods Scientifically Proven to Prevent and Reverse Disease, Michael Greger MD with Gene Stone (Pan Macmillan, 2016)

The Power of Meaning: The True Route to Happiness, Emily Esfahani Smith (Rider, 2017)

Thrive Fitness: The Vegan-Based Training Program for Maximum Strength, Health, and Fitness, Brendan Brazier (Da Capo Press Inc., 2009)

Acknowledgements

Love, gratitude and appreciation to the team at Hay House for extending me this great opportunity: Michelle Pilley, Amy Kiberd, Elaine O'Neill, Zoe McDonald and Julie Nolan. Special thanks to Michelle Pilley and Amy Kiberd for supporting and encouraging my journey from day one. In helping me to spread a message of love, health, kindness and compassion, you gave me fulfilment in being an ambassador for change. Thank you for your patience, your kindness and your support. You believed in me when I hit rock bottom and lost faith in myself. For helping me find my way back to the light, I thank you.

To my nearest and dearest Myla-Grace, Adonis and Nico O'Holi, Malaika Cherie Bolatiwa, Michelle McCarroll, Makella Benjamin, Monique Reed, Nathan Reed, Derek Reed, Gloria Reed, Beata King, Michael Burchadt Nu Bodhi, Violetta Isolde Aurora and Shaa Wasmund.

Thank you for your love and support throughout writing this book and my journey into veganism.

ABOUT THE AUTHOR

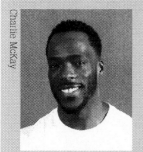

Charlie McKay

Edric Kennedy-Macfoy is an ex-firefighter, a fitness coach and a vegan. After experiencing the loss of more than 10 family members and close friends to cancer in a short timeframe, Edric began to seek out answers on health and decided to adopt a vegan lifestyle.

Now retired from the London Fire Brigade, Edric runs boot camps and fitness programmes that help people stay fit and healthy. He believes his mission is to help those in need and to change lives for the better. He is the author of *Into the Fire: My Life as a London Firefighter.*

 Edric Kennedy-Macfoy

 Edric_KM

 @Edric_KM

 EdricKennedy-Macfoy

www.edrickm.com

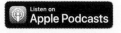

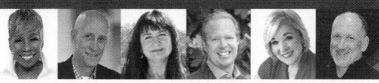

HAY HOUSE

Look within

Join the conversation about latest products,
events, exclusive offers and more.

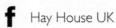   Hay House UK

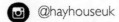   @HayHouseUK

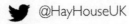   @hayhouseuk

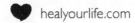   healyourlife.com

We'd love to hear from you!

Printed in the United States
By Bookmasters